Conception Diary:

Thinking About Pregnancy & Childbirth.

Dr Susan Hogan

The work was first published in the U.K. in 2006 by:
Eilish Press
4, Collegiate Crescent
Broomhall Park
Sheffield
S10 2BA
England.

ISBN-10: 0-9551656-0-1
ISBN-13: 978-0-9551656-0-3

British Library Cataloguing in Publication Data
A catalogue record for this book is available from the British Library

Library of Congress Cataloging in Publication Data
Conception Diary: Thinking About Pregnancy & Childbirth/ Susan Hogan.
p. cm.
Includes bibliographical references and index.
1 Women's studies. 2. Pregnancy & childbirth.
3. Conception-infertility.
I. Hogan, Susan, 1961-.

This book is dedicated to Robert

Acknowledgements

Unreserved thanks to Teresa Barnard for her editorial and encouragement. Teresa is a talented academic and writer and surely has more important things to do than trawl through my material, so thank you for this act of friendship Teresa.

I would like to express gratitude to the au-pairs who helped create a little writing time for me, and most especially to Maristella who was fun to have around and to Annie who has just joined us.

I am indebted to Michael Lindley of the *Truth Studio* for the front cover design.

Conception Diary: Thinking About Pregnancy and Motherhood.

Tuesday 25th February 03.

Today I experienced dotting in front of my eyes, which then intensified and turned into blurry vision. My first response was terror that it might be an aneurysm, a tiny brain haemorrhage which might forever alter my life. After seeking out the campus 'first aider' I found myself in an ambulance, for the first time, being cheered up by a genial and handsome medic. At one point in our conversation, I suggested that he must have saved some lives in his time but he responded ruefully that he "lost more than he had saved" after which an uneasy silence ensued.

Casualty was a salutary experience. I sat watching people whose normal lives had been ruptured, disrupted (as mine had just been) by a variety of misfortunes from heart attacks to car accidents. Most lay in beds, which appeared to have been scattered around the large room in a haphazard manner. A few sat crumpled on chairs; virtually none were speaking. Most were lying or sitting in their beds looking bewildered, wired up to machines; others were wearing oxygen masks. Some were alone; others were accompanied by distressed, blank-looking, or, in a couple of cases, weeping relatives. One elderly couple wore a resigned look of those who had been through this before. It occurred to me, for the first time, that this might be something to be endured many times over – the reprieve, before the end.

Everywhere there was activity, with oxygen cylinders being wheeled about and beds moved, bells ringing, and all the time a steady stream of new admissions disgorged from ambulances, then hastily surrounded by a team of medics.

What all of the disparate humanity in the accident and emergency ward had in common was that we were all waiting to be trolleyed off into the bosom (or perhaps the bowels) of the hospital to be saved…. Yes, to be saved. That's what it felt like.

Although my ovulation had not yet occurred that month, I knew that sperm could lurk about for some time (hardy things apparently) so I had counted last night's love making as my first attempt to get pregnant. The thought suddenly seemed bizarre in the setting of the hospital emergency room. Would I still be able to have a baby? What was happening?

Eventually, I was given some tests and as my symptoms had vanished I was sent home. I was feeling too tired and stressed to want to have sex that night. It seems hard to think about giving life to others when one's own suddenly seems in jeopardy…

Wednesday 26th Feb 03.
Another day followed of tests at the hospital. They think it's a virulent virus, so nothing too serious to stop me having a baby. Nothing to stop me having a baby – it's taking a while for the words to sink in.

Thursday 27th Feb 03.
Tonight when we were having sex I looked into Robert's eyes and wished that the sex would result in a baby. We are feeling so tender towards each other. Robert is *desperate* for me to conceive.

Friday 28th Feb 03.
Today I was flicking through a copy of the Times Higher and became mesmerised by a large colour photo of an eight-week-old foetus, floating disembodied in what looked like the cosmos. The head and eyes looked like that of an alien – the eyes the wrong shape and hugely out of proportion with the tiny head. The body was a little pink mass with peculiar little deformed-looking limbs protruding from it, but the extraordinary thing was that there were individual-looking fingers. Yes, I'd seen these sorts of photographs before, but I'd not really seen how astonishing they are.

Saturday 1st March 03.
We had sex at night and again in the morning. Clearly, we are taking this seriously!

Sunday 2nd March 03.
I keyed in 'determining the sex of baby' on an Internet search today and ended up in the Harvard University Medical School Consumer Health Information site, where there was an article by a Robert Shmerling MD. It suggested that sperm carrying Y chromosomes swim faster, but do not last as long as their X carrying counterparts. Therefore, sex at the time of

ovulation privileges the faster Y carrying (male) sperm; however, if sex occurs a few days before ovulation the 'male sperm' die out leaving the 'female sperm' advantaged. Visiting another site this information was repeated but in a way slightly less flattering to the 'male sperm', which were described as weaker, smaller and less strong than the 'female sperm'. Another site suggested that 'male sperm' and 'female sperm' prefer different amounts of acid or alkaline in the vagina. But, frustratingly, the piece did not go on to suggest ways of influencing this through douches or diet.

I realised that all this frequent sex prior to ovulation was giving the advantage to X-carrying (female) sperm.

Later, Robert gazed so lovingly into my eyes as we had sex that night. He hasn't said so but I know he wants the 'conception sex' to be really lovely.

Monday 3rd March 03.

Over dinner, my three women friends seemed entirely uninterested in the topic of how to influence the sex of the baby so the topic was quickly dropped. I was told I was "mad" to want to have a third child (this said by a woman who has three herself). The conversation turned to episiotomies, induced labour (how the contractions are particularly painful because of induction) and Caesarean Section. With eight children between us, only one of the births had been relatively painless and free of medical intervention…

Tuesday 4th March 03.

When I told one of my best friends over the phone that I was trying for a third child she absolutely screeched with amazement, evidently, I'm not seen as the maternal type! She is 20 weeks pregnant, just recovering from having had amniocentesis and had been feeling really ill for three days, she told me. Having received contradictory information from blood tests and a scan result, she had been strongly pressurised, she had felt, into having amniocentesis, which is invasive (and I'd always imagined rather painful as the needle goes through the woman's stomach into the amniotic fluid). It carries up to a two per cent miscarriage rate (some sources say 3%), but as she really didn't want to risk having a *Down's Syndrome* baby she felt she had to take that risk.

She asked me about my experience of having had ‘amnio’ and I corrected her that I’d had CVS instead (partly out of cowardice because there is no needle through flesh involved, but I didn’t say that).
I was surprised that she didn’t know what CVS is (Chorionic Villus Sampling) because she’s an avid reader and so I assumed she’d have ploughed through lots of books and researched the topic of pregnancy thoroughly. The technique called ‘placental biopsy’ entails a sample of the placenta being analysed. A hollow needle is inserted into the uterus via the vagina and a small amount of placental tissue (Chorionic Villi) is sucked up through it. A scan shows the position of the needle so that only placental tissue is selected. During my last pregnancy, I read a lot of literature on CVS, which may be associated with low birth weight babies. Furthermore, if performed early (before ten weeks) some literature suggested links to high rates of miscarriage (up to 4%) as well as foetal abnormalities caused by the test.
So, most of the phone call was spent explaining CVS and catching up on her work. I’d been saving baby clothes for her, because I knew she was ‘trying for a baby’, as the expression goes, but (hopefully) I’ll need to keep them for myself now.

Wednesday 5th March 03.
My boyfriend’s sister, Katherine, sent me an article she’d seen in the London Standard *‘My Baby Diary’* by Lucy Cavendish. In this, Lucy described meeting her midwife for the first time and being given lots of contradictory information about blood tests, scans, diabetes and amniocentesis. Furthermore, she was told that she’d have to book all her own appointments including her appointments with the midwife (I quite like that idea as I would prefer to be prodded about less than previously, but I can also see that it’s daunting). When Lucy asked questions she was given yet more printed information. When she asked about different local hospitals she was told they were all much the same. “How does anyone know what to do and where to go?” she pleads at one point in the conversation (prior to bursting into tears), to which the midwife retorts, “It’s called patient choice”…

Thursday 6th March 03.

Well, I think I've ovulated already, but I suggested that Robert and I have sex "just in case", to which he replied, "I'd got it into my head that I could have Thursday and Friday off". Clearly, I am wearing the poor man out.

Friday 7th March 03.

Well, I could be pregnant now – just a matter of waiting…

Saturday 8th March 03.

I was tempted to pop into the baby clothes section of a local shop but I managed to restrain myself. I bought myself three new dresses instead, though I'll only get to wear them for about three months if I am pregnant.

Sunday 9th March 03.

I did another internet search and found a site which suggests vaginal douches for determining the sex of the baby. So it was a tablespoon of white wine vinegar in warm water to preference 'female' sperm. I'll try it next month if I'm not already pregnant. Having just had a boy I'd really like to have a girl.

Monday 10th March 03.

When I was sitting in the bus this morning a dignified-looking African woman boarded with a tiny bundle of a baby tied to her back. She sat opposite me but I could not see the merest trace of the baby's skin so tightly was she pressed against her mother's back. The mother rocked back and forth almost imperceptibly and the baby was soundless. I found myself beginning to feel anxious that the baby could breathe. I looked more closely but could not get a glimpse and my sense of anxiety intensified until it became discomforting.

I remembered when I used to carry my daughter, Eilish, in a baby sling hugged close to me but I was always sure that I could see her little face. When she was new-born I would feel compelled to check her basket when I couldn't hear her breathe. In the end, it was easier to have her in my bed at night where I could always hear that she was alive, still with me – miraculous though that seemed when she was so vulnerable-looking, so tiny. It didn't help me to get a good night's sleep though.

Tuesday 11th March 03.
Today I did a chalk drawing of the foetus I hope I have inside me. After I'd done it I felt quite protective towards the little sketch, which had become talismanic in some way.
Later, I wondered why I hadn't depicted the maternal-foetal unity? Why had I depicted a disembodied foetus? Perhaps it's just because we are so bombarded by these strange and beautiful images of motherless foetuses, foetuses that seem to have an independent existence.

Thursday 13th March 03.
My period, earlier than usual, started at work. I'd been so convinced that I was pregnant I hadn't packed any tampons and I had been so engrossed in work that I hadn't noticed until I'd gone to the loo and by then I was covered in blood. It was the first time I'd really thought about the blood symbolising the loss of something, a possibility of another life disappearing in the blood.
And I was surprised – really surprised. As my boyfriend had managed to get me pregnant twice before whilst using contraception I'd begun to think of him having SUPER SPERM. It hadn't properly occurred to me that conception might not be instantaneous. So I ended up thinking for the first time about the possibility of not having another child and felt choked, now that I have a vision of three.
I see the two little ones sitting on a rug in a puddle of sunlight in our garden surrounded by toys. Their older sister is overseeing them and I am there just to pick one or another up to cuddle or feed or change. I am relaxed and contented.
This I know is not a very realistic picture, as my real role will be to arbitrate and protect. Emile (now fifteen months) won't sit still for a moment and he will be forever ranging into the flowerbeds and tearing up clumps of plants. His older sister, Eilish, (nearly six) will retrieve him repeatedly, patiently, but a little too roughly, so that he will end up screaming and complaining – besides he wants to destroy the garden, not sit peacefully with us. When he is brought back to the rug he will attempt to bash his newborn sibling (a name for which I have not yet found) with a heavy toy. Only my quick intervention will prevent injury – thus I will not be able properly to relax or read. Eilish will demand to hold the baby

and manhandle it (I imagine a girl baby though she will be dressed in her brother's male-coloured cast-offs, thus always confusing people's reactions in public places). I will be tense and alert, ready to catch the baby should Eilish drop her on her head, or ready to break her fall should Eilish trip. Every now and again, Eilish will get bored with trotting off to fetch Emile, so I'll have to take my turn too. This will get tedious after a while, as I do not share my daughter's patience in performing repetitive tasks. When Eilish and I attempt to play a constructive game (as we will at some point), somehow Emile will sabotage it by trampling on the board, cards, and pieces. Simultaneously, the baby will start to cry for a feed. And that's what it will really be like, endlessly, endlessly.

Friday 14th March 03.
I wanted Robert to hold me in his arms. I wanted to weep while he held me for the little foetus we don't have. That might sound utterly histrionic but it occurred to me that we might never have another. I am forty-two.

Saturday 15th March 03.
Today Robert said something negative about my appearance, and I responded with a savage ferocity out of keeping with the remark. My pent-up emotion unleashed itself. Furthermore, I want to feel adored by the man who is making me pregnant. **Adored**. I felt upset by the distance he must have been experiencing, which allowed him to make the remark. He has allowed himself to feel close to me whilst trying to impregnate me, but as soon as my period started he becomes remote and critical. I wondered if it was an odd sort of narcissism allowing his intense love for me only when I am a container for part of him, or a potential container. I am not sure if I should have this man's child and yet I feel pain at the thought of not having it.

Sunday 16th-Thursday 20th March 03.
I have been ill with a virus. First Emile had it and then me. (Fortunately, Eilish, whose sixth birthday is on Saturday, seems fine). I've had a fever and spent all of yesterday in bed. Despite the fact that it's a wonderful sunny day, I'm about to go back to bed again. Robert said last night that he thought it was good I wasn't pregnant because he'd have been sick with

worry about the foetus (and the possibility of a miscarriage) with me so feverish. I know he's still angry about my outburst on Saturday, but I wish he'd feel concern for me. ME. I'm too ill to think straight, but I can't imagine us trying for a baby again this month; I feel too angry about his distance, his lack of concern for me.

I stumbled out of bed not knowing how yesterday's vote in Parliament had gone and shuffled into our lounge to be confronted by images of Baghdad being hit by cruise missiles. I was utterly stunned both by what had happened and by the detail of the images. You could almost see individuals dying – well, not quite, but it will be possible soon.

Reality has turned into one of those games played obsessively by ten year olds, except it's the cradle of civilisation being hit by rockets and real mothers and children being randomly blown up. Yet we have 'smart bombs', bombs which can hit targets with great accuracy using satellites, so this was a policy decision to murder with impunity.

I had read in *The Guardian*, a reasonably reliable paper, that often more civilians die in such conflicts than armed military personnel. I know that 'we' have been killing their children for a decade through sanctions, but I couldn't help looking at my little 15-month-old baby tottering around, unaware of the horror depicted, and wondering how many more had been killed by the cruise missiles.

Friday 21st March 03.

I read a line in a book today which made me pause and think: 'Acquiring and then tending – these eat up women's creativity, anyone's creativity.' I know this applies to possessions but what about children? Will my tending eat up my creativity?

Today, feeling a lot better, I walked in the sunshine in the local botanical garden. Emile was wearing his first proper pair of shoes and holding my hand, walking unsteadily in the unfamiliar garb. He looked so joyful that everyone who passed us smiled at him or both of us (including two male police officers), something I find quite strange, as I am not immensely extrovert.

Emile was in ecstasy fondling different plants, fingering dead leaves, running his hands over tree bark, chewing pampas grass, smiling. And I was sharing his moment of awe of being in the jungle of plants, excitedly

watching squirrels. Surely his being there enhanced my perception, helped me to sit longer, look more carefully, enjoy more fully…?
And from the park we go to the school to collect Eilish and her friend Chloe for a birthday 'sleepover'. I wonder to myself if I wouldn't prefer to do this than work and delegate the care of my children to others, which is what I so often do.

Sunday 22nd March 03.
On Saturday our au-pair arrived. My life is about to be transformed. No more snatched moments at the pc with Emile at my feet with his little pile of toys; however, this morning she was unpacking so I tried to write, but he was not prepared to look at his books depicting ducks or other babies, or play a musical instrument – his glockenspiel is his current favourite. I'd done a little percussion session with him to put him in the mood: tooting on the recorder, shiggeling the rainmaker, tapping the drum, shaking the tambourine and maracas. I'd saved producing the most wanted glockenspiel to the moment I sat down at my desk (yes, clear tactics). Nevertheless, as soon as I sat on my chair he came over to complain so I turned my computer off and went to him.

Monday 23rd March 03.
Maristella, our new au-pair, has gone up even further in my estimation because she appeared to be amazed (or at least feigned surprise really well) when I told her I was ten years older than my partner, Robert. Later, I discovered that she had told Robert he looked twenty-six at most, which delighted him and puts me at around thirty-four or five!

Tuesday 24th March 03.
Time to start trying for a baby again. We need to have lots of pre-ovulation sex, to preference the 'female' sperm and also to lower his sperm count which also preferences the production of 'female' sperm, I read somewhere. We were more passionate than loving last night, but I don't believe the conception sex will influence the baby's personality!
Must start using the douche in a couple of days… I ovulate on Friday, I think, though my cycle varies slightly from month to month so it's possible that it might not be until Sunday. Will use the douche from

Thursday to Sunday – must remember. I do really want another girl.

Wednesday 25th March 03.
Today I did another drawing. I'd intended to depict the foetus but I ended up producing a rather abstract picture of a woman's swollen belly and breast in profile; however, there was no womb or foetus – though the picture felt more resolved once I'd added a suggestion of a womb. Having decided I want another baby I do see my body differently now. The picture felt unresolved because that's how I feel. I don't see my body as simply my body, but as potentially fecund. On the other hand, I don't want to see myself as failing if I don't conceive. It mustn't become my *raison d'être*. I've started preparatory work for a new book even though I know I won't finish it if I get pregnant again as I can't write academic work when pregnant (something to do with the brain shrinking, or exhaustion, or both…).

Thursday 26th March 03.
I found myself telling someone today that I was hoping to have another baby; however, I heard myself also calmly telling this person that at forty-two I was by no means convinced that I could conceive again. She in response told me that she has many friends and acquaintances in their forties either "desperate" to get pregnant or newly pregnant. She, at forty-five, believes that her decision not to have children is final, though she wondered if she is "missing out".

I suggested that having children or not having them is like playing a musical instrument, or not playing one (I always feel the need to try to say something comforting). To play an instrument really well, to have mastery over it, must be profoundly emotionally satisfying. But we who don't play an instrument don't spend our time wandering around worrying about not being able to do it, do we? We don't fret, "I'm forty-five and I still don't play the violin…" or "I'm nearly 40 and I haven't mastered the cello…" Perhaps people who have such talent pity those of us who are musically mute, but I didn't articulate that possibility. I don't pity childless women. Not having children is merely the absence of something.

Bernadette and I have had several of these sorts of conversations, because she knew me before I had my baby son, Emile. At that time she was thinking of having a baby. Her husband would have to reverse his vasectomy. She would have to change the life-style she enjoyed.

Such conversations are slightly awkward, as I never know what to say in response to childless women's regret. On another occasion, I explained, "It's just another relationship isn't it?" – and suggested that I experienced my relationship with my daughter as an intense relationship – as intense as that with my 'husband' (she seemed surprised by this). Now the relationship is here I can't imagine not having it; I value the intense love I feel. But, as with any relationship, we have difficulties, which have to be resolved. I spend a lot of energy in this relationship and because she is a child, my daughter, I must do this even when I'm not feeling like it. But that's no different from having a husband, is it, I reason? You may be tired and want to be alone, but you'll probably talk to him when he gets home before you slope off… It's just a relationship that has to be sustained.

So not having a child is simply one less intense relationship. But I know it's more complex than that even as I say it, because women are seen as naturally maternal and because the nature of the relationship with a child is different to any other. My daughter's love is intense and almost unconditional. When I get home at the end of a working day it is she who throws herself, with abandon, into my arms.

Friday 27th March 03.

I take my multivitamin with folic acid (essential for the development of the baby's spinal cord) and wonder if there is any change in my body. No, I don't feel pregnant. Last night, before sex, I used my vinegar douche and again this morning; however, I'm about to go swimming and wonder about the effects of chlorine on the lurking hardy 'female' sperm. I imagine chlorine is not very good for sperm in general, especially lounging round in the jacuzzi, as I am wont to do late on a Friday afternoon. It is a shame if my attempts to keep fit undermine my attempts to get pregnant. I must ask a friend, who is a chemist, if my swimming will harm the X sperm.

I wonder if I should buy a home ovulation test. I can tell, more or less, from the position of my cervix when I am ovulating. Also I become more interested in sex at this time of the month. Indeed, today is the day according to my calculations…

I remind myself to enjoy not being pregnant. I have lots of energy at the moment and soon, if this pregnancy is like the last two, I'll be feeling tired, mentally sluggish and slightly nauseous. Time will slow down so that the nine months will feel more like two years! I will enjoy not being pregnant – today's mantra…

Saturday 28th March 03.

I have started working on my new book, which will explore the links (or postulated links) between maternity and madness. It's going to be called *Maternal Discourses.* I came across an 1895 quote by the psychiatrist, Henry Maudsley:

'…there is nothing nice in the process of parturition nor in the base services which the child exacts'.

I guess the 'base services' include nappy changing as well as feeding. I remembered just how lovely it was breast-feeding my children, especially when they were newborn and fragile. There is one particular image which I treasure of Eilish lying asleep on my naked belly. It's one of the things I'm sure I'll enjoy the third time around too, if I conceive again.

Newborn breastfed babies produce faeces which smells of milk, so it's not until solid food is introduced that it starts to smell bad. I get used to the particular smell of my own baby's shit, but faced with someone else's baby, yes, my stomach does turn. But Maudsley regarded baby care as degrading and the 'fuss' surrounding it to be irrational since the baby is merely an 'excretory product': that's right, he uses the word 'product'; the baby is not even regarded as human. By implication, women who indulge in this 'fuss' are irrational since they have these bizarre emotions for the 'excretory product'. Yet we do have this link that causes our breasts to swell with milk as the baby calls out, and we do, many of us, delight in the new life we have created which seems more miraculous than anything else… But giving birth and motherhood still seem to be degraded in our culture… What has changed since Maudsley's time? That's what I intend to find out.

Sunday 29th March 03.

When you are a mother, you always have to trade off one thing against another. I am not with my children. Admittedly, I attempted to find them

in our local park, after viewing a house for sale (of course we need a bigger house). I couldn't find them and I felt sad because it's a beautiful sunny day and I can't think of anything I'd rather do than be with my children in the park, in the sunshine. It's what we did last Sunday. A perfect day with Robert, Maristella and I taking turns to look after Emile, who is going through a demanding phase. Taking turns to just to sit in the sun, read the newspaper, supervise and play. But today I couldn't find them. We'd viewed two houses in the morning *en-famille* and decided that I'd view the third on my own. Emile squeals like a pig about to be slaughtered every time we try to contain him or strap him in his car seat at the moment, hence the idea of viewing the third house without children. So I get to sit at my pc, but knowing that I'm missing out.
I wonder if I am pregnant yet? I don't feel different. I don't feel suddenly and inexplicably exhausted or labile. Now I must wait. I want a baby girl…

Wednesday 2nd April 03.
I haven't had any time to think about whether or not I am pregnant. I am not feeling pre-menstrually tense, so therefore must be pregnant. I am feeling tired, so therefore must be pregnant. I felt slightly queasy this morning, so therefore I must be pregnant; however, I am feeling libidinous (I often experience a surge of sexual interest before a period), so perhaps I am not pregnant.

Thursday 3rd April 03.
I am feeling emotional. Sitting at a table on a packed inter-city train I pick up *The Guardian* newspaper and read: a van packed full of Iraqis, mainly women and children, has been fired upon at a US checkpoint in Iraq killing ten. The report quoted Mr Hussan, a survivor interviewed at his hospital bed, who told the reporter that 11 members of his family had been killed: his parents, two older brothers, their wives and two nieces aged 12 and 15, his daughters aged two and five and his son aged three. 'His wife, Lamea, who is nine months pregnant survived. Lamea said 'she saw her children die.' To watch your children die - I tried to visualise the scene of blood, panic and shock and I found myself in tears, crying for Lamea and her lost children, for their crumpled, bleeding, broken bodies.

Even as I write this, my eyes prick with tears to imagine the mother's pain watching her children die. The British are inhibited. At least if you cry in public everyone pretends it's not happening, so nobody asked me what was wrong. Perhaps I am labile because of the row I had last night with Robert. He withholds affection as punishment. It's a little tactic of his, part of his regime of control. I, on the other hand, get cross.

Yesterday I was feeling fragile, for no particular reason, and I wanted his attention, if only briefly. I wanted him to hold me. I tried to get his attention, unsuccessfully. Part of the problem is that we have children – he cooks, he cleans, he fills the dish-washing machine. Today I drop him at the supermarket, because he doesn't drive (and won't learn), as it's his turn to do the fortnightly shopping. I help Eilish with her homework. I put her in the bath and read her bedtime stories. I tidy and pack for my trip. I fold clothes and put them away. He watches television whilst playing with Emile: we are all activity. It was the same last night. I am not cross but I display a flicker of exasperation. Though I regain control immediately it is enough for Robert to be irritated and want to punish me. I have transgressed. I have displayed emotion inappropriately. (He is a right-time-and-place-for-everything kind of a man. Discussions of arguments normally go with his saying something like "Well, what you should have done is…" Or "What you should have said is…" and then he'll formulate the sentence that would have produced a positive response from him). So, anyway, later when finally we are in bed together he refuses to hold and comfort me. When I react he says that he "would have fucked me if I hadn't 'huffed' earlier". He tells me (infuriatingly) what I should have said; however, the damage, it appears, has been done and nothing I can say now can ameliorate the situation.

He seems unaware of my fragility or perhaps he does not care how I am feeling – or perhaps he is angry, but does not talk about his feelings.

Later, I tell him that I have decided to use contraception again until things are better between us. I want us to be close and harmonious while trying for a baby. I want to be heard. I want him to take my needs seriously even if they cut across our bloody routines. I need the man I am trying to have a baby with to care about me, to be caring. He ends up responding angrily that he "won't fuck me if I use contraception". We have reached a new low. I am angry and sad. I hope I am not pregnant.

This morning, Robert took me in his arms and apologised for not 'hearing' me, for not being more sensitive. He held me in his arms while I cried silently. Momentarily, I think things will be fine.

Before I left for work my fifteen-month-old baby, Emile, threw himself into my arms when I held them outstretched and demanded, "cuddle". I kissed him and held him and chased him all round the house. When it was time to leave, I wished I could stay with him so we could go to the park in the sunshine.

Today I hope I am pregnant. I sit on the train and blink back tears for Lamea who has only the child she is carrying inside her left in her devastated life.

Friday 4th April 03.

I wake up feeling slightly queasy. Am I pregnant? Waiting to find out feels so hard, but soon I am too busy to think about it.

Later, in bed, I read another sentence, which gave me pause for thought. It was the assumption, often expressed by friends and relatives, that the author of the piece would move cities to be with her long-distance boyfriend, rather then the other way around. She wrote: '…but almost no one asked if Doug planned to move to New York. It was frustrating how people expected me to radically amend and truncate my life so it would fit comfortably into his.' It was the phrase 'radically amend and truncate my life' which caught my attention. This was precisely what I had done, am still in the process of doing. Can I fit comfortably into Robert's life? I am beginning to have doubts.

I had been a single parent since Eilish's birth (indeed, my marriage had been utterly on the rocks at the time of her conception) and I made the decision to go ahead with the pregnancy anyway, but demanded nothing of my ex who has no regular contact with us. I met Robert when Eilish was almost four. (Most people we know in Sheffield assume Robert is her father, and of course he is – though not her progenitor). When I got pregnant again, I took the decision to have the baby regardless of what happened to my relationship with Robert. Actually, I took the decision not to have an abortion which is slightly different if I think about it. The relationship flourished. When a school place became available for Eilish last December I moved, away from my academic job in another city, over to Sheffield to be with Robert and for us to be a family. So I write this having only lived with Robert full-time for three months – and yes, we are having some teething problems.

Robert is very domesticated and does most of the work around the house (it's his house so he is used to looking after it). Nevertheless, being here forces me to make a long and stressful commute to another city for my work. I am now thinking of applying to work part-time. Indeed, the commute has made my full-time job feel untenable. People are suggesting that I should ease up on my research activity (the most satisfying bit of the job). I seem to be the one making all the compromises, all the changes. And I am truncating my life. I am writing less. I am not attending conferences, or giving papers, or seeing friends – Robert has given me a little desk space in the bedroom, which is literally just big enough for my p.c. He has given me this and one cupboard, into which I must cram everything…

Saturday 5th April 03.

Today I read another disturbing piece in the newspaper. It is about another US checkpoint incident in Iraq; however, this time a suicide bomber kills several people. The strange thing about the report is that in the car there was a heavily pregnant woman. The report read: 'A pregnant Iraqi woman stepped out of the car as it approached the checkpoint and began "screaming in fear", US military officials at central Command in Qatar said. Moments later the car exploded, killing three soldiers as well as the pregnant woman and the driver. Two American soldiers were injured.' The woman may have been forced to go to the checkpoint, the piece speculated. Or perhaps she was a suicide bomber who just lost her bottle at the final moment? But, if that were the case, why didn't she attempt to run away from the car if she knew there was a bomb in it? Perhaps she was walking along the street and abducted at gun point – perhaps when the car stopped at the checkpoint she had a sense of what might be about to happen, an act of violence of some sort, but not sure of precisely what – hence why she just screamed and didn't run? Perhaps we'll never know what happened.

Tuesday 8th April 03.

I have been very very busy, which prevents me thinking about my attempts to get pregnant; however, in bed I checked the position and shape of my cervix. I seem to have less fluid retention than is normal at this time of the month. Also I am ravenously hungry (though this can also be a reaction to stress. I have the urge to eat when work upsets me, as it almost always does these days, because of the departmental in-fighting). I lie in bed and hope that it is not my imagination that this month I have conceived.

Wednesday 9th April 03.

Yesterday I saw a job advertised I think I could have walked into had I not met Robert, had Emile and tied myself down to Sheffield. He won't consider moving. The choice I have made is still sinking in. I suppose if I'm pregnant starting a new job is a silly idea; however, it's a senior position to the one I have here and in a city I prefer, with lots more money and better conditions. Yesterday, I felt that having another baby was far more important than anything else. Today, I feel frustrated at having my choices so limited.

Thursday 10th April 03.

My period started and I feel gutted. Even though I'd love to apply for the job advertised, and I have contradictory emotions, I clearly am very emotionally tied to the idea of having another baby.

I just can't imagine being a full-time mother; however, being an academic in another city full-time isn't working. Although I have a good working-at-home agreement, envious colleagues often seek to undermine it – well, one in particular, as I can get dragged in for important meetings and this… [my editor has insisted I remove the expletive that I'd wanted here] often arranges important meetings on my working at home days – especially meetings which particularly demand my presence. This is despite my explicit requests that she not do this. I sometimes expect this kind of behaviour from those childless women who haven't grasped what motherhood is like, but this woman has had children. This is just nasty. I am beginning to detest women who power-dress, grow testicles and act with complete insensitivity, at best. (Perhaps she has just assumed a corporate mentality which is thoughtless and heartless; I'd prefer to believe it wasn't malicious).

Yes, I'm moaning; however, Wednesday, (my most contested working at home day), is the one day that Robert can't collect Eilish from school, so I do it. Why not send the au-pair? Well, we don't always have an au-pair, so none of our routines can depend on having one; moreover, the school is miles away (the local school was full so we took a place out of the catchment area for this address) so it would be an excessively long walk for an au-pair (and I always worry that they will become unhappy if asked to walk too much in our terrible British weather), whereas I can pop up in the car in five minutes. The child minder is even further away (she was the most local we could find) so I normally collect Emile in the car at 5.30pm. When I can't do it Robert has to take a taxi. So, as you can see, there is lots of disruption to my family's routines every time this happens and for what? I sit in these, often very unproductive, meetings resenting every second I'm there.

I'd like to drop down to a small fraction (a fifth at most) but I can't get paid maternity leave if I do this, so I'm feeling torn by my conflicting impulses to get out (so that I can spend more time with Emile while he's little, be around to help Eilish with her home-work more often) and stay and get supported maternity leave (which I feel I'm due because I've worked really hard for the University and feel I'm owed this). And of course there is no certainty that I will conceive again.

***

I had a lovely time bathing the children, playing with Eilish, helping with her homework, cuddling her. She is affectionate and funny and I love being with her in the evenings. After she goes to bed I get to spend time with Emile. Last night I was lying in front of the fire building tower blocks for him, which he gleefully knocked down – over and over again. In the background was a video of this week's *Late Review*, but I didn't get to hear much of the cultural debate over his squealing. He is also keen on passing things back and forth. He can say "mama", "no", "her" (which is said whilst he makes a beckoning gesture with his hand, so is supposed to be 'here') and "night night". He can climb up and down the stairs. The most important thing about Emile is that he is very charismatic. He finds most things funny and has a beautiful smile and a happy temperament.

Friday 11th April 03.
Both of my regular soaps are featuring maternal themes. In *Friends*, Chandler and Monica are babysitting Emma who is Ross and Rachael's baby. Rachael informs them that Emma is "pooing" a lot and screams every time her carer disappears from sight. Looking after a baby is not being portrayed as much fun. Even Joey, who is not renowned for his sensitivity, comments on Emma's crying all night. Nevertheless, Rachael does not look tired and has had time to put on full make-up, comb her beautifully conditioned hair etc. (of course, this is fantasy: the actresses never appear without full make-up). As a concession to motherhood she has appeared in a couple of episodes in a frumpy smock, which hid her breasts. At least Rachael can bear to leave Emma now… There had been an absurd scene a few episodes ago in which Ross's mother is obliged to sit at the bar of a restaurant with baby Emma so that Ross and particularly Rachael can keep an eye on her whilst eating – clearly the Rachael character demonstrated that she has the requisite maternal impulses.
After Ross and Rachael are off the scene, Chandler and Monica decide they want to have sex but not in front of the baby. Of course, the scene is played for laughs but it is clear that neither character could feel comfortable 'humping' in front of a new born. Even when baby Emma dozes off they go to the bedroom rather then having sex in the lounge where the cot is. Furthermore, they agree not to make too much noise! There is an underlying assumption that Emma might be psychologically damaged in some way and/or that it is perverted to perform in front of a baby (even when it's sleeping). There are often highly conservative undertones in *Friends*.
In *Sex in the City*, Miranda has just decided to go ahead with her accidental pregnancy. She is not in an ongoing sexual 'relationship' with the father (it was a one-off "fuck" with her ex-partner – indeed, a "mercy fuck" as she was feeling sorry for him) she figures that as a thirty-five-year-old single woman she may not have another opportunity to have a baby. (I made a similar decision in similar circumstances at the age of thirty-seven). Although the narrative in *Sex and the City* is self-consciously radical and provocative, there is a reactionary undertow. Miranda's decision is in part prompted out of fear that she might end up like Charlotte who has just been told by a fertility advisor that she has only

a 15% chance of conceiving, and who is absolutely distraught because she really wants a baby above all else. So the biological clock is ticking at the back of the plot.

Another conservative aspect of the script (introduced by Carrie's boyfriend, Aidan) is the suggestion that men have a right to know about conception, even in the case of casual sex resulting in pregnancy where the woman decides to have an abortion. This is reinforced by the fact that Steve (who has just unknowingly impregnated Miranda) is a highly sympathetic character. (Miranda says things could hardly get any worse without her having to confront Steve's feelings about it…)

Aden's suggestion, that men have a right to know, is highly problematic as it could put American woman at risk of litigation, or even violent responses from men they hardly know. This ultra-conservative stance is not really rebutted in the plot but slightly fudged when Carrie implausibly meets the boyfriend who had made her pregnant many years ago, and whose foetus she had aborted without telling him. When he fails to recognise her she reminds him of their date. He cannot remember their having had sex. The plot ends with a remark that men are sometimes lucky not to know.

Saturday 12th April 03.

I have spent so much of my life feeling afraid of pregnancy it's strange to now long for it so much. Before I became pregnant for the first time I absolutely dreaded what it would be like. Something like a bad 1950s science fiction movie in which I'd be taken over by some other being. Or like *Alien* in which the thing lodges in John Hurt's stomach only to burst out in the most dramatic of circumstances, destroying him in the process. But the foetus did feel like part of me (though I wish that Eilish hadn't decided to do quite so much thrashing around in the middle of the night). Because of the womb squashing other internal organs, particularly the lungs, as it expands it is hard not to feel compromised. Your body is designed to give life to the foetus and that may be at some cost to you.

I read yesterday that Mary Wollstonecraft, the author of *A Vindication of the Rights of Woman* (1792) who is often trotted out as a founder of modern feminism, died at the age of 38, from puerperal fever following the birth of her daughter Mary (who was to become Mary Shelley, incidentally). I am grateful for modern medicine. It made me remember how many women in the third world die following childbirth because of infections or whose children die for want of clean water (diarrhoea is still a big killer and entirely preventable). Although I plan a home birth, I know that all the resources of modern medicine will be there if necessary, especially antibiotics.

Tuesday 15th April 03.
I have been very mummy so far this holiday. Today I spent hours in the park while the children enjoyed the slides and play frames. Emile mastered a small slide and a tunnel as well as enjoying pushing his buggy around. Yesterday we went to a wood and then on to a playground. Both children were much admired. Someone asked where I'd got Eilish's shoes (big pink over-the-top flowers with cloth petals on a sandal, which she'd chosen herself). Two people commented on her dress and three women flirted with Emile. The day before that we all went to the botanical gardens and I spent lots of time with Emile who wanted to caress trees and pull at shrubs while Maristella and Eilish raced about on a high-speed tour. I enjoy being with Emile on his own – the slow pace is peaceful.

Now I get to do an hour of intellectual work. "Would you like to do an hour of intellectual work before dinner?" offers Robert. I accept. He thinks I'm working on my other book – the one that will bring me kudos and career advancement.

Eilish, my six-year-old daughter, has begun to flounce off in a 'strop' whenever she perceives she is being criticised. Sometimes she misinterprets a conversation which is playful and light-hearted. I suppose this is a 'developmental stage' that psychologists have written about but I feel disinclined to dip into that literature. Today she came to me whingeing because she thought she was being criticised "for not looking after her legs". Robert and Maristella had been remarking on her bruises and cuts (quite an impressive array) from her frequent falls. She came to me snivelling and I convinced her that watching a video in Maristella's room with bunny, her favourite toy, would cheer her up.

Robert arrives on the scene and tells me she slammed the door. I laugh as I find her emulating adolescent behaviour, seen on children's TV, quite funny. He smiles and I think everything is OK. But it's not, as he has already told her she can't watch a video in Maristella's room. I suggest she does. He says no. I back down, even though I'm thinking that he is being unreasonable and that, if in a high-strung mood, she is better on her own. I have a little talk with her and offer her three choices – felt-tips with mummy upstairs, playing in her room, or video with Robert, Emile and Maristella in the lounge. She chooses the latter and disappears downstairs. I think that everything is fine. But it's not okay, as Robert has decided that, even though he didn't ask me, I should have produced a firmer response to Eilish's outburst. He rejects me when I try to give him a hug and makes a hurtful and hostile remark. I lose my temper with him yet again. Happy families…

Now, reflecting on it, I just feel profound sadness that I am unable to second-guess his demands and that he is so unable to express what he wants from me. I'm also disappointed with myself that I end up yelling.

Sunday 20th April 03

In episode 12 of the soap *Sex in the City* ('*Just Say Yes'*) Charlotte and her partner, Trey, are having a traumatising time having unsuccessfully tried hormone treatments, presumably injections of Clomid or Pergonal to increase her production of eggs, (which may be linked to quite dramatic increases in ovarian cancer). She wants to start IVF. They have become a "barren couple" (a phrase that recurs during the episode), though she also uses the phrase "reproductively challenged" at one point. Her husband refuses IVF because of the low success rate and invasive nature of the treatments. He is exhausted. She screams at Trey at one point (the hormones are making her aggressive) that she feels as though it's she who's doing all the work: taking the pills, having the hormone shots, talking to all the other 'reproductively challenged' women in her building and chat room, learning Mandarin (in case they adopt a Chinese baby), doing the research, whereas all Trey has to do is "jerk off into a plastic cup"!

To add more stress to their situation, his mother makes clear her disapproval of their considering adopting a Chinese baby girl. The mother's response is both sexist and racist because only a blood-linked male heir will do.

Miranda, who got pregnant accidentally, tells the progenitor, Steve, because she feels he ought to know now she's decided to continue with the pregnancy – though she makes it clear she does not require his support, saying that it is just something she wants to do for herself, "It won't be your problem," she asserts. She's a well paid lawyer so can make such an assertion. (Miranda slept with him once because she had been feeling sorry for him, following his operation. Steve, it may be remembered, has only one testicle following treatment for testicular cancer). His initial response on hearing that she is pregnant is the quintessentially male, "I guess it's good to know my one ball is working".

Later he turns up at her apartment and when Miranda opens her door there he is on bended knee with a ring in outstretched hand. "What are you *fucking crazy*?" retorts Miranda. They will not marry because they are having a child. Miranda is having a tough time with so-called 'morning sickness' and is vomiting "all fucking day". (We do get to see her vomit but she nevertheless looks quite glamorous). I was lucky I was never afflicted with sickness, morning or otherwise, during either pregnancy.

In *Friends* there is a hilarious scene in which Chandler and his wife, Monica, talk at cross-purposes. Chandler thinks Monica intends to have a boob job (a lie told to him by Joey) and keeps telling her how perfect her body is and how he wouldn't want it to change. In particular, he wouldn't want it to get any bigger. Monica doesn't know anything about the boob job lie, so she thinks he is talking about their forthcoming pregnancy and that Chandler is freaked out at the prospect of her body changing shape. She tells him that her arse will be getting bigger too. He is horrified by the idea of her having an arse enlargement. Then Rachael and Monica point out that her hands and feet might get bigger too, not to mention the loss of bladder control. Chandler is perplexed. It's a very funny scene and he doesn't twig they are talking at cross-purposes until Rachael demands angrily how he'll cope at the hospital with the blood and the screaming and "the little person shooting out of her". As an after-thought, Rachael adds that it is a magical time…

Monday 21st April 03.

Although I'm looking forward to having another baby, I can't say I'm looking forward to being pregnant again. I was so exhausted during my last pregnancy, but I was a single parent then, so being able to rest more often might make a difference, though there is still the problem of my job – even though I'll take maximum maternity leave this time (if I don't quit before I conceive), it's still a slog trying to lecture whilst pregnant. I felt queasy for at least the first ten weeks during both of my pregnancies. It's quite hard to feel so ill for so long. Then later, there is that urge to nap in the afternoons. Once I nearly crawled under my desk at work as I felt I couldn't stay awake. Then much later there was the feeling that I was about to explode – that I would give birth *any moment*. Though I was nearly two weeks early with Emile (hence his birth in the back of a black cab while the birth pool bubbled away unused in a different city), *I couldn't believe he hadn't arrived earlier*! In fact, I can hardly believe I'm going to go through all that again.

I forgot to mention Emile's birth. I guess it's time…

Picture Robert and I sitting talking animatedly in the back of a black London-style taxi. We are on our way to a neighbouring city where the birth pool and midwife await us. Our 'birth partner', Nadine, had just boarded a train from Edinburgh and had promised to phone us from Newcastle to see how we were getting on. It starts to snow.

Now imagine a spine-chilling scream! In a state of disbelief, I shriek for the driver to take us to the nearest hospital. I fall to my knees gripping the handles in front of me and scream, 'Arrrrrrrr!' repeatedly. I can no longer talk, only shriek. We had just reached the Bramall Lane roundabout in Sheffield as Emile appeared, delivered into Robert's arms, after just a few massive contractions. I am in such a state of shock I do not move. I remain rigid, on my knees, until we reach the hospital. I suppose the location was rather ignominious but there were moments of beauty: Robert wrapping Emile in a T-shirt and hugging him to him as soft flurries of snow enveloped the taxi. This is my overriding image of the whole event.

We did look like a case for accident and emergency rather than a maternity ward when we arrived at the Jessop Hospital for Women. Robert was drenched in a mixture of blood, amniotic fluid and vernex. I was still on my knees, transfixed… They cut the cord while we were still in the taxi (no opportunity to negotiate a natural third stage!). I was wheeled in a wheel chair and I was in such a state of shock I did not object! Fortunately, I managed to expel the placenta as soon as I started moving about. Emile was whisked away to an incubator, not because there was anything wrong with him, to warm him up, as it was a chilly day. We were at home (Robert's house) later that day, after the paediatrician had performed the routine checks and I'd filled in a mass of forms. Robert's parents, Jacquie and Rumy, surprised us by turning up at the hospital unannounced and then posing as a taxi company! (Obviously Robert had rung them earlier). The Muslim taxi driver, who had been driving throughout, told Robert it was one of the most wonderful experiences of his life!

When we went to register Emile's birth a few days later, the woman at the desk proclaimed, "This is interesting, I've never had an in-transit before." Robert says that from first contraction to babe in arms it took 1 hour and 25 minutes.

Tuesday 22nd April 03.

I know the precise moment in which I realised I wanted a third child. It was a glamorous occasion – the launch of my third book, which took place at the former home of Sigmund Freud, the famous Viennese psychiatrist, in North London. I was introduced to a child psychologist I hadn't met before. We chatted for quite a while, both slightly tipsy from the wine. Although I had never contemplated having a third child, when she told me she had three I felt a surge of envy. I tried to dismiss the feeling. I did the usual rationalisations: we'll never have a child-free holiday again as none of our relatives would take them all; it would be more difficult to find au-pairs and baby sitters; we'd never have an uninterrupted night's sleep again; one of us would definitely have to work part-time (this was before I was seriously contemplating part-time employment); because I'm the only driver I'd be constantly dropping off and picking up; we'd be poor. But that was it. That was the moment. I was rather hoping for reviews or better still a TV slot, but that was the only important thing to come out of the event, for me at least.

Wednesday 23rd April 03.

I hadn't seen Robert for several days. One of the first things he thrust at me when he arrived in Edinburgh was an article from *The Observer* on the Fertility Awareness Method (FAM, for short) popularised by someone called Toni Weschler. Having practised natural birth control more years ago than I care to remember (before AIDS reached my consciousness and condoms became the birth-control method of choice) I was aware that there is an increase in body temperature following ovulation. Pre-ovulation temperatures vary from 97 to 97.5. Post-ovulation, it rises to 97.6 to 98.6, so said the piece. But that's not much help because by the time the temperature changes it's too late to conceive (though it's good for avoiding conception or for knowing when you can give your husband a rest); however, plotting the graph for a few months can help to identify precisely when ovulation occurs.

I'll consider plotting my graph if I don't conceive in the next three months. I think I know when I'm ovulating as I experience heightened sexual interest, my cervix is soft and open and I am wetter. It is the time of the month when *I must have sex.* Still, there's no harm in double-checking if it doesn't happen quite soon. Day sixteen is O DAY, I think.

Thursday 24th April 03.

This is definitely spoiling my enjoyment of sex. We are both feeling under pressure. Even though this is my receptive time of the month, I just haven't been really responsive. I announced that I'd rather we relaxed and just had sex when we are in the mood, even it means we have to wait longer for conception. Perhaps I'm just tired from working so hard…

Friday 25th April 03.

In *Sex in the City, 'The Good Fight', episode 13* of my favourite soap Miranda, who is pregnant, has sex with a good-looking older man (who is not the baby's progenitor). She worries that this is "tacky". At one point, prior to the date, she wonders if a big dick could harm the baby. Miranda is a sassy, intellectual character and we imagine she knows the answer to the question – what she really wants is encouragement from her friend Carrie about the date. She regards this flirtation as her last chance to have sex before the bump starts to show. It is inconceivable to her that someone might wish to have sex with her once she is obviously pregnant – one taboo which a series, that sets out to be challenging, might tackle.

Meanwhile, Charlotte and Trey have given up trying to have a baby – or at least they have given up trying by artificial means as Tray has refused IVF. She is distraught, whereas he is trying to get on with life, and have some fun. His attempts to cheer her up are gauche in the extreme. Clearly, she is not going to accept being childless, while he feels that she is enough for him. Their sumptuous apartment and his high income are not solace for Charlotte (who has given up her own job as an arts administrator to be a mum). The increasing acrimony between them is highlighted. When he, inadvisably, gate-crashes her "girls" night dinner party they clash in front of the others; and when he objects to her mentioning his erection problems in public, she retorts that they all know about his flaccid penis already, and that they are sick of hearing about it! Trey is mortified. The marriage, it seems, is doomed.

Saturday 26th April 03.
The job I haven't applied for closed today and I hope to God that I won't end up feeling resentful about not being able to apply for it. Robert won't move. I probably wouldn't feel so bad about not applying if I were feeling more positive about my current employment (now I've moved to Sheffield I find the commuting stressful). He says he doesn't know anyone in Edinburgh. I point out that I know nobody in Sheffield and that his job is more mobile than mine. I also point out that he has no close friends in Sheffield, just acquaintances, that everyone close to him is in or near London. He points out that Edinburgh is further away from London than Sheffield. I suggest that my Edinburgh friends would become his – he thinks not, and besides "they are all at least ten years older than me". I can't be bothered to remind him that I am ten years older than him and that this does not seem to pose a problem. I point out that what I do is more specialist and that it's a much more competitive field with less openings and that it would make sense for him to support my career by moving. And round it goes.
It looks as though I'm going to drop down to a fractional post and spend more time with the children. I hope I'll be able to adjust. I hope I'll be able to get to feel at home here in Sheffield. I have thought of leaving Robert but I can't do it. The only decision I need to make is whether or not to take a paid maternity leave first - on that point I am indecisive and, in any case, I'm still not pregnant, as far as I know.

Sunday 27th April 03.
Robert dropped what feels like a 'bomb shell' on me to-day. Although his "vision of the future" until recently always contained an image of three

children, suddenly he has started visualising "only the four of us", (I want to query the absence of an au-pair, who would make the total five, but restrain myself from interrupting) and he feels this is okay. He went on to elaborate that although he'd be "utterly delighted" for us to have a third child, he has realised that it might not happen.
This left me feeling slightly bewildered as I had felt *very* under pressure by Robert to have a third child and I do really think there is nothing more important; however, the reality is that children are tiring and demanding and that the tiny bit of space and time I have to myself will shrink to nothing if we have a third (not to mention feeling exhausted for a year: nine months during pregnancy and for at least the first three months).
We have been having sex every day. I like sex but feeling under an obligation is putting me off. Normally, at this time of the month I am very responsive, but the last three times it has felt mechanical and I have felt emotionally disengaged. I thought it would be *sexier* trying to get pregnant.
I guess with the Iraqi invasion just having drawn to a grisly close, I shouldn't use expressions like 'bomb shell'. Although the war is officially over according to the invading coalition, *The Observer* newspaper today had a heart-rending picture of a burnt baby screaming on its front cover. An arms dump, perilously near to civilian housing, blew up sending a Fog missile into the nearby community, killing at least twelve and injuring many more. The newspaper suggests that this incident may further heighten hostility towards US forces among ordinary Iraqis – as if relations could deteriorate much further…

Monday 28th April 03.
Sometimes I love being with my children more than anything else. Other times I feel I'm going through the motions. On Friday I spent two hours going through a backlog of homework sheets with Eilish. How did we get so far behind? (The guilt of a working mother is endless, being on holiday I have been trying to make up for never spending enough time with her). Each of the homework sheets has a maths and English question and then two from science, art, music or R.E. They are fun. To give an example, one of the P.E. questions was: 'put your hand on your heart before and after you jump 20 times. What happens? Does it change?' And a music question

was ‘put different amounts of water in three bottles and tap them with a teaspoon. Listen and discuss the pitch’. Luckily, I enjoy this sort of thing, though getting her to memorise the spellings of new words is less enjoyable.

Anyway, on Friday I loved every minute of it. This Sunday, finishing off the sheets, my patience was tested. Now why should I love one session and not the other?

For the last hour she’s been making a plasticine “museum” and I’ve just been summoned to buy some items so I should go…

Tuesday 29th April 03.

I looked up FAM (Fertility Awareness Method) on the internet today. Although ovulation varies from woman to woman, we tend to ovulate about 14 days before menstruation. The egg lives for only one day and sperm live for only three to five days (I thought they could last longer). Conception it likely to occur on the day of ovulation or in the 4-5 days prior to it, so says the Brown University site.

In an article by Elizabeth Anne Arnon M.D., on another site, she discusses how to feel your cervix. Basically, it feels soft and open, rather than hard and closed, during ovulation. Cervical ‘mucus’ varies too and is altered by changes in hormones during the monthly cycle. I don’t like the word ‘mucus’ so I’ll refer to ‘juice’ – sounds much sexier. Our juice becomes more plentiful towards ovulation and then slightly sticky in the most fertile period. Dr Arnon tells us to look out for viscous juice, which is like ‘egg-white’ and is stretchable.

Having looked at my own cycle, I can see that my judgement of my ovulation time was good. In my standard 28/29-day cycle (counting the first day of bleeding as day one) I’ll ovulate around day 14/15 and should be having sex from day ten through to day sixteen and perhaps to seventeen for luck (in case of late ovulation)! So FAM has made me realise that although I was roughly right about my ovulation time I’d thought I was fertile for longer than is actually the case. Given that I’m starting to suffer from intercourse fatigue, this is useful information that will allow us to have sex at precisely the right time next month – if I’m not pregnant already, of course.

Must get to work on my book *‘Maternal Discourses’,* which is what I should be doing right now. I haven't much time, as on Wednesdays Robert can't collect Eilish from school at 3.15pm so I must watch the clock.

Thursday 1st May 03.
Barbara looked at me with an expression of triumph. "What are your needs?" was her question. My needs seem so varied, so contradictory, that I faltered and shrugged. "You see", she beamed, "you don't know what your needs are – you don't think about yourself". Clearly, Barbara felt she had accomplished something of a coup by elucidating this part of my personality, so I felt sorry to disappoint her by pointing out that I think about my needs all the time. The trouble is their irreconcilable nature. I also knew in that moment that she does not have children. (I did a mental check: no playthings in the garden, no small shoes in the hallway, no clutter in corridors). If she were a mother she would know the visceral sense of being torn in many directions all the time.

If only I could devise strategies for 'meeting my needs' more often. If only I could enjoy, guilt-free, my time-out away from the children. If only I could sit at this p.c. and not remind myself that Eilish's home-work sheet needs attention, that I must ask Robert if he has a puncture repair kit for her bicycle tyre, that I must phone *Scallywags* to check if they have a slide in stock, that I must send a cheque for her French club, buy her chalks as promised, check their hair for nits, buy Emile new shoes – the list goes on. I haven't even looked at the laundry basket or the state of her bedroom – those things really don't trouble me. Indeed, 'remind myself' is too active a description of what happens. These things just pop into my head and distract me. I shoo the thoughts away but they buzz around like mosquitoes on a warm summer's evening.

"Why are you thinking of having another child when you are already overstretched?" she later asks in the same session (my second, and probably last, therapy session with her). I respond by saying that, yes, children are demanding and tiring, "but that having children just feels more meaningful than anything else." She looks at me blinkingly with a slightly startled expression. She doesn't get it. Of course she can't get it.

There is a huge gulf between those who have children and those who have not, but it's only those who have crossed over who are fully aware of it. I cannot talk to Barbara about my needs or anything else I feel. "Yes, I must chill-out more," I say… But what I'm thinking is, 'I can't talk to a childless person about my wanting to have another child. I don't need therapy; I need more time just to be alone: just to be…'

Tuesday 6th May 03.
My period started and this time I didn't feel devastated. In fact every month feels like something of a reprieve – another month in which I'll have enough energy to work on my new book and enjoy my children without getting exhausted. I'll be quite happy if I don't conceive until the autumn.

Wednesday 7th May 03.
We've decided to stop having 'trying to have a baby' sex. Last night I had the most enjoyable love-making I've had with Robert all month. We both knew I couldn't conceive at that point in my cycle. Even if it takes us longer we have agreed to just have sex for pleasure, which will mean having less sex during my fertile phase. It could mean that we don't have a third child, but at least sex won't become a chore.

Thursday 8th May 03.
I guess some people reading this will think, 'Why does she want a third child? She could simply have more (so-called) quality time with the two she has?' My response is, 'Absolutely, I think that myself all the time'. Why not spend more time with my existing children? That would be an utterly rational thing to do, and if I can't conceive it is precisely what I will do. But I haven't mentioned my miscarriage yet. I had one in December and no it wasn't a big trauma because the pregnancy was unplanned and it happened early. Nevertheless, there is a *crazy, irrational* part of me, and *I do realise that this is mad thinking*, which thinks that that foetus, which didn't make it, would like to have life. Or to put it another way, that foetus showed us that it is possible for me to produce more life – an idea that hadn't occurred to us before then, at least emotionally. Prior to the miscarriage, we were feeling grateful that I had been able to have a 'trouble-free' pregnancy and healthy baby age at the age of nearly 41.

Friday 9th May 03.

I had a long chat with Becky on the phone, as it's her 39th birthday today. She is six and a half months pregnant and has very high blood pressure. Concern has been expressed about the possibility of her developing pre-eclamsia (a build-up of fatty acid in the placenta which can undermine its function) and she has already given up hope, it seems, of having anything approaching a natural birth. She says she has been "passed from pillar to post", being told, on the one hand, that she must have total bed rest and, on the other, that she must attend this or that appointment (requiring a walk to the hospital, as she says it's impossible to park there, which sends her blood pressure into orbit). Once there she is passed from one professional to another, which she finds stressful and annoying (not helpful for keeping her blood pressure low). On a recent visit, having been thoroughly messed around, she sat waiting to see a consultant for over two hours. There have been scares too: on one occasion her blood pressure was so high she was sent immediately to hospital and ended up hanging about on a maternity ward. She hasn't seen the same person twice throughout her pregnancy. When I expressed dismay about this she merely replied, "Well, this is London, isn't it…?"

I was quite shocked by all this drama as Becky was salsa queen prior to her pregnancy and is very fit and healthy and was (prior to pregnancy) quite slim. She is also very assertive and I'm sure that if anyone could extort a good service out of an overburdened and crumbling NHS Trust or local council, she could. Indeed, I am utterly convinced that the service must be dire. She feels that even though her pregnancy is 'high risk', there is no one overseeing her care.

I'm sipping my first Gin and Tonic of the weekend and lounging about rather than having my Friday late afternoon fitness session and suddenly I'm filled with guilt that I'm not looking after my body well enough. I'm more than three years older than Becky and my last pregnancy was only relatively problem-free because I was very, very fit.

Saturday 10th May 03.

My six-year-old daughter, Eilish, told me with no forewarning, "Abby's baby has died". When I asked who Abby was, she explained that she is a girl in her class at school. "Abby's baby died, not today but on another day," she repeated. "Abby isn't back at school," she added after a pause. I clarified that it was Abby's mummy's baby – "she stopped breathing – a teacher came in and told the class." I don't know what it was – perhaps the simple way Eilish told me – but I nearly burst into tears.

Sunday 11th May 03.

In my soaps the maternal themes continue – well, sort-of. In *Friends* the baby disappears quite conveniently. Neither storyline concerning the parents (Ross's visit to the country or Rachael's flirtation with Joey) contained either the baby or reference to the baby. A few episodes ago Rachael couldn't let little Emma out of her sight – now she doesn't give her a second thought. The baby was absent in last week's episode, but a reference was made to the parents giving up the use of expletives.

In episode 14 of *Sex and the City*, entitled *'All that Glitters'*, Miranda is asleep when the girls call to ask her out. She is "always" asleep. Indeed, she is sleeping away her last months of "freedom", we are told, prior to entering the prison of maternity - not a great advertisement for becoming a mother. Miranda goes to a gay nightclub, *'Shirtless Heaven',* with her girlfriends. She bumps into a male colleague from her law firm. He is embarrassed. He's not exactly in the closet, he explains, but he wouldn't want the senior partners at their firm to know that he's gay. She reveals that she is pregnant. She, in turn, asks him to keep quiet about her pregnancy or she'll no longer be allocated the best cases and have colleagues vying for her office.

The following day Miranda is seen confronting this colleague for blabbing about her pregnancy. He exclaims that he was defending her as she'd been spotted lying asleep under her desk several times and was suspected of having an alcohol problem. Her retort was that being pregnant in a conservative law firm was considered worse that having a drink problem. Meanwhile, Trey and Charlotte decide to separate. She says she feels like a "bad person" for "needing to have a baby". "I don't think I should have to give that up" she says tearfully to Trey, who had refused to continue having IVF, or to adopt a Chinese baby. Her friends support her by saying that she is entitled to her "needs". The subtext is that it's a biological impulse at work, which Charlotte is right to yield to.

Monday 12th May 03.

The World Health Organisation has decreed that women should breast-feed for the first six months, Louise informed us. A long conversation ensued. I didn't ask how old Sarah's baby, Vandon, is but she is about to give up breast-feeding (I think he is over six months). Apparently, he can get distracted and bite. Although Eilish, my first born, bit my nipple a couple of times, I screeched so loudly that she soon got the idea this was not a welcome activity; however, if babies fall asleep on the nipple, sometimes they clamp with their teeth. Vandon does this and so did Eilish and I remember having to stick my little finger in her mouth to prise it open. Sarah had already discovered this technique.

Louise didn't like breast-feeding. One of her babies, Leah, refused to take a bottle but she felt she had done quite well to have managed three months with each of her other two daughters. She said she had a very determined mid-wife, otherwise she might not have breast-fed at all. I talked about feeling on my own. It had never occurred to me that I might have problems breast-feeding. After all, you simply stick the nipple in the baby's mouth and they suck – right?

Eilish was a 'natural' home birth and I had planned that her suckling my breasts (following her birth in the birth pool) would stimulate *oxytocin*, a chemical that helps the body to expel the placenta; however, when it came to it she didn't want to feed and I ended up having to march around and squat and grunt in an undignified manner to get the placenta out (a process which was also excruciatingly painful as I had torn slightly). Eilish was self-sufficient. Indeed, Eilish didn't want to feed until my breasts had turned into two rock hard bazookas. And although I had read in a book that newborn babies don't always want to feed and sometimes they are not hungry for days, I hadn't realised that I'd end up in agony and that my breasts would be leaking all over the place. As I write, I remember the very distinctive smell of newborn milk mingled with fresh blood (the girl baby also produces blood from her vagina, strangely enough – something to do with the cocktail of chemicals swirling around in her system). Then, eventually, when she wanted to feed, she had difficulty latching on to the nipple because my breasts were so full and rock hard and she got frustrated. There was a lot of screaming, I recall.

I vividly remember being utterly alone with my screaming baby and

enormous, uncomfortable breasts, weeping inconsolably.
Then, when Eilish did feed, I was surprised at how it stimulated uterine contractions which were quite painful and which produced more blood. She would only feed on one side (the nipple being a slightly more congenial shape to her) so the other breast continued to leak.
When my mid-wife blithely talked about me milking myself and freezing the excess milk I wanted *to murder her* as my breasts were not amenable to being 'milked', even though full. I had tried the technique she had showed me. I had bought a breast pump, which seemed to draw only a miniscule amount after an eternity of pumping. (And you can't read a book while pumping – it's boring).
Things changed. I ended up feeling totally relaxed about breast-feeding and fed my first for an unfashionably long length of time (almost until school, though towards the end it was just a bed-time feed) but as a single parent there was just me and her – no male in the picture pressurising me to stop. She still nuzzles up to my breasts for comfort and says she can remember suckling. I digress. I felt at ease about breast-feeding in the end, and fed Eilish (and later Emile) on packed intercity trains, park benches, buses, inside shops, in the children's section of *Waterstones* bookstore (which had a no breast-feeding policy at that time, and perhaps still does, though I was never challenged); I used to sit on one of those little children's seats and feed her. Louise pointed out that we still don't see many women feeding in public and she's right; we should see women feeding all over the place…
Anyway, because it ended up being so easy (no messing about with bottles allowing spontaneity) sometimes I can forget that it was hard at the beginning; however, it never occurred to me not to feed. I have a stubborn personality.

Tuesday 13th May 03.
Can't help myself, but I have been counting off the days again. This weekend coming is my fertile weekend.

Wednesday 14th May 03.
I saw my father today. This is a rare event, so worthy of mention. He is a very shy, retiring man and rather socially inept (in sharp contrast to my

former in-laws who are both socially skilled and good raconteurs). He lives a long way away and remarried shortly after my mother died of cancer. I don't think my daughter recognised him so he had to announce that he was her grandfather. Except when I picked them up and plonked them in front of him, he hardly related to the children, but he had a couple of spurts of energy in which he seemed interested in me... though he then drifted off into a reverie.

The evening was a great success. There were no rows and Emile was the centre of attention, dribbling a football up and down their big kitchen and firing goals at uncle Allan. I had the longest chat I'd had with my niece, Beverly, for ages, which I was pleased about. Eilish had a ride on *Strawberry* the pony. My sister's new stallion, which charged back and forth and ran up to the gate at which he was standing, entranced Emile.

The evening was significant in reminding me, very forcefully, of the tensions within my family. Robert sulks every time my in-laws are mentioned, even though they have agreed not to mention Eilish's progenitor (their son, my ex-husband, with whom she has no contact). I understand that Robert wants to be Eilish's father. I want Eilish to have a father. I believe that she will have a better life if Robert loves her and does not treat her radically differently from his biological child, Emile. Eilish was only three and a half when they first met so should be able to bond with him, I reason. I don't want to jeopardise this and yet I think she has a right to see her other grandparents and they have a right to see her. I like my in-laws. ('Ex' in-laws, strictly speaking).

My father's partner, Joan, started a conversation off by asking about them. She is verbose; a torrent of infinite nothings gushes forth. Joan, incidentally, is a former friend of my mother (I loathed Joan as a child). Robert fell silent and sat looking stormy. I said that Mary had come to my book launch in February but that I hadn't seen her since. Robert shot me a look. Well, I had to answer the question, hadn't I? I steered the conversation elsewhere but I felt sad I couldn't talk freely. Mary has asked for Eilish to visit but I know as soon as I broach the subject it will cause a row. Being stubborn, I will insist that she visit them and Robert will be cool and distant with her on her return – perhaps for weeks. And I don't know what to do or what is the right thing to do. I wish he'd be more rational and realise it's in her best interests to continue to have a relationship with them, but evidently he can't be.

Friday 16th May 03.

Today when I arrived at Emile's childminder no one answered. I knocked harder. I waited in case she was in the bathroom. Eventually, I tried the front door and it opened. In the hall were a small baby and a child who I guess was about three or four – both completely unattended. I asked the older child where the childminder was and he replied, "sleeping". I should have asked "does she do this often?" In the lounge was the slumped body of the child minder and she didn't stir when I said her name. *I actually had to shake her to wake her up*. I left my son with heavy misgivings. Once in the car, I phoned Robert's mobile and left a message on his phone saying I wanted to find another childminder.

Later, after I collected him, we returned to an empty house. Maristella, the au pair, was still nowhere to be seen (she was supposed to collect Emile). Clearly, she has forgotten that she is on duty from 1.30pm on Fridays. Lucky that I'm working from home today, otherwise on my return from work there would be umpteen disgruntled messages on the answering machine from the childminder about Emile having not been collected.

Well, I better do some marking while Emile is having his afternoon nap since I am officially working at home today.

Saturday 17th May 03.

In episode 15 of *Sex and the City,* in an episode entitled *'Change of A Dress',* Miranda is wondering when her 'maternal gene' will kick in. Looking at an ultrasound scan of her baby leaves her cold and when the technician tells her excitedly that "it's a boy" – she fakes a pleased response. And it is the first of several such faked responses. Indeed, she has started worrying about herself – ultimately civilisation may be at risk, she muses.

So there is Miranda drinking salsa (a non-alcoholic drink) and wearing a dress with an elasticised waist. It's not until the baby kicks her that her emotions are stimulated.

The following episode (16), entitled *'Ring a ding ding,'* had Miranda, heavily pregnant, big, 'gassy' and 'swollen' (and breaking wind uncontrollably). Her fingers are fat. Even her feet are fat, so she has to buy new shoes. Her "ass" is also big and she regards herself as undesirable – indeed, "unfuckable" (That's why husbands are a good idea, because they are obligated to continue to have sex during pregnancy, she quips). At one point she calls herself ugly – not a good message for pregnant viewers.... When she gets together with the baby's progenitor, Steve, to work out a care schedule for their contract she asks him to fuck her, as all she can think about is sex. She has become the "mercy fuck" now. "This doesn't mean we're a couple," she warns him as they make out. The voice-over tells us she had multiple orgasms – lucky Miranda.

On *Friends,* which I am watching concurrently for contrast, as it's a soap about young people, rather than people of roughly my age (the actress who plays Samantha in *Sex and the City* is five years older than me) the emphasis is back on sex. Rachael's baby was nowhere to be seen again. Although it doesn't pretend to be a realist comedy (the main actors are all so stunning they could be professional models), there does seem to be a dichotomy between the smocked and, to my mind, quite unsexy mummy figure of Rachael (who worries about swearing or talking about body parts in front of her baby) and the Rachael who is at the roof top party being "slutty" and wanting to get laid.

Sunday 18th May 03.

Robert decided to pleasure me in other ways last night so he could save his sperm for tonight. I'm away in another city on Monday, on day 14 of my cycle, and back on Tuesday (day 15) so he wants to give me his sperm as a going away present to take away on my trip.

*****

It was a rainy Sunday afternoon so a good moment to get out the plasticine. Eilish and I made highly decorated cakes for the cake shop and then took turns in buying and selling them (she makes up all the rules).

We then took Eilish and Emile to the Asian supermarket shopping. Emile looked so sweet tottering about holding Robert's hand. Even some young lads at the bus stop smiled at him.

Emile is nearly seventeen months old now and he has a sweet repertoire of little noises: "yea, ya ya, wah wah, bah bah, da", " il y a", and my favorite: "mu mu mu". His only really distinctive words are "night night" and "here", though he does greet me with "mu mu". I'm wondering how he'll relate to the baby. Robert says he visualises the three children together "all the time" but I must admit I don't. I tell Robert I'd be worried about Emile, who is now a strong and robust baby, biffing the newborn with a chunky toy…

What is that cliché about motherhood being good for stimulating capacities for 'multi-tasking'? I'm writing this while Emile puts different shoes on my feet and then takes them off – over and over again. He is a shoe fetishist (I hope he'll get it out of his system at a young age - better to indulge him, I reason). I'm not exactly Imelda Marcos but I do like shoes. Emile has selected the most sparkly and outrageous and has been putting them on and taking them off – but he's very young, so needs assistance. I type with legs prone to make it easier for him…

Now he's decided to chuck them all down the stairs one by one (over the stair-gate) – that will allow me about 10 minutes of being able to type in a normal posture! I do like the iconoclasm of babyhood…

On second thoughts, perhaps I'll just go and play with him…

Monday 19th May 03.

Well, it never occurred to me that this might be a dangerous thing to do; however, I've just read an article from the *The Observer* in which a columnist, Lucy Cavendish, admits that she has been threatened with physical violence because of her views on parenting. Lucy has been writing for the *London Evening Standard*, which I can't get here in Sheffield, about having a baby and dealing with the NHS. It seems her column has aroused much controversy from all quarters. Talking about the excruciating agony of her drug-free home birth brought her into conflict with supporters of natural childbirth, who suggested that home births might decrease as a result of her negative column. When she wrote about feeling exhausted, disillusioned and having difficulty enjoying her newborn baby, she received hate mail. When she wrote 'I feel guilty, stressed and exhausted so don't bully me into breast-feeding for six long months' she received criticism from the breast-feeding lobby. When she admitted to having her baby in bed with her after drinking alcohol, she received more hate mail. Clearly, the personal is very political when it comes to parenting. On the other hand, she says that she has received lots

of supportive mail from women who found the adjustment to motherhood very hard.
Lucy accuses mothers of being 'paranoid' and as not sufficiently trusting their 'instincts'. There is little room for the 'Natural Mother' in the midst of all this politics, she concludes. Well, I suppose it's not surprising she's feeling a little defensive.

Wednesday 21st May 03.
Robert and I had a row and ended up not having sex on Sunday night after all. I was away on Monday (day 14 of my cycle) and when I returned on Tuesday Robert announced that he had thrown away all my contraception. His reasoning was that if we had a row I couldn't start using it again if it wasn't there. I'd been so cross with him on Sunday that I'd filled myself up with spermicide, just in case any of his sperms were lurking around ready to impregnate me. I'd regretted the gesture as soon as I'd calmed down.
I made the point to Robert that it would be better not to row in the first place rather than to throw my contraception away. He had said that my using contraception was "irrational", but I felt the opposite – that is was entirely rational not to want to conceive with him when he was being unkind to me.
We ended up having sex and as it was day 15 of my cycle so I might have been ovulating. I did my douche first to preference the 'female sperm'. We'll probably have sex again tonight – day 16, just to be on the safe side.
Off the subject of sex, I just went out and bought a Barbie bike with stabilisers for Eilish and an interactive beetle for Emile. The beetle has buttons on its back which, when pushed, make tropical rainforest noises. I think it's really sweet. I also bought various odds and ends which will make suitable gifts for children's parties. I am avoiding working on my other book, the serious academic one. The reading I have is on Victorian murderesses: I'm researching infanticide and Enlightenment philosophy as the backdrop for looking at 19th Century psychiatrists' views on motherhood.

Thursday 22nd May 03.
Eilish was delighted with her new Barbie bike and we had to do a little run

on it before the rain set in. It was such a pleasure seeing her so happy. She is very easy to please at the moment.

I wish my relationship with Robert were so straightforward. He doesn't like the way I communicate with him. I don't know what it is exactly, my tone or posture – he can't pinpoint it except to say I seem agitated. (On one occasion it was the look on my face – I hadn't said a thing).

So today I said, "What's going on?" and that was enough for him to be hostile. What happens after his initial expression of irritation is that I then get upset or more agitated and so he makes barbed, snide or supercilious remarks. I then move from being slightly affronted, upset or frustrated to feeling angry.

"Why were you hostile?", I demand. "Because you irritated me," he responds. "Why get irritated when I definitely wasn't angry at that point? I'm sure of it. I just came in to find out why we weren't doing what we said we'd do." "You just irritated me"– and round it goes.

He says it's nothing to do with his need for control. He just *needs me* to "behave myself". In other words, to behave in exactly the way he'd like me to behave if he were able to control me.

I guess lots of people would like their spouses to behave in certain ways, but there is something about his immediate expression of irritation which is punitive. It's like a slap. I didn't meet his expectations so I've got to change, otherwise I am punished. I've got to adapt to how he'd like me to express myself. There is **no question** of him changing his communication style, learning to respond without irritation to my intensity, *hearing what I'm actually saying and responding to it.* The latter really does seem like too much to ask for: to actually accept what I'm saying at face value.

He says " I get under his skin". I retort that he merely seems not to like me very much. He refutes this – and round it goes. He says I overreact; however, from my point of view, I could be somewhere else. I don't have to be here. *I choose to be here.* Perhaps because I'm older and I've lived abroad in the past, have had more relationships, I really can imagine having a different sort of life. If he won't treat me with respect then I don't want to be in this – that's how it makes me feel. When I try to articulate this feeling, he accuses me of "making threats". And I do end up making threats because he has taunted me.

I feel after this last argument that I want to stop trying to have a baby. I didn't articulate this, but I feel I have raised expectations about the quality of our relationship because we are 'trying to have a baby'. We might be more relaxed together if we stopped trying for a few months. I've just ovulated so I've got a month to think about it.

Friday 23rd May 03.

In *Sex and the City*, in an episode entitled *'A Vogue Idea',* (I hadn't noticed that all the episodes have naff titles until I started writing this) Miranda is persuaded, by the ultra broody Charlotte, to hold a 'baby shower' in Charlotte's luxurious apartment as a way of getting all the things she needs for her baby. This is strictly a women-only event in which the mother-to-be is showered with gifts which she opens in front of her guests so that they can be admired, so that the generosity and taste of the giver can also be appreciated. The absurdity of some of the items given is neatly satirised and Miranda shows a total lack of interest in the infant entrusted to her at one point during the proceedings.

I often get the impression that *Sex in the City* is written largely by men (note to self: I must check this). Who do you invite to a baby shower? "The bitches" who invited you to theirs, offers Samantha, who articulates much of the misogynist discourse in the series. Indeed, Samantha is all male fantasy – the women who always looks gorgeous, who will fuck for hours and always wants to give 'head' and, here's the real giveaway – she cares about the size of a man's dick. Only men care about the size of each other's dicks.

Prior to the big event, Miranda has a *contretemps* with Charlotte about her lack of preparations for the birth (psychological and practical). Of Miranda's perfectly ordinary apartment Charlotte, who has been obsessing about becoming a mother, exclaims, "This place is a death trap!" And has Miranda thought everything through? For example, has she given proper consideration as to whether to be a "marsupial mum" or a "stroller mum" (can't one be both?) or where to put the crib? Perhaps Miranda is intending to sleep with her newborn? Miranda responds, "Can't I go to jail for that?" (Sloppy script-writing, as she is supposed to be a sharp lawyer, or perhaps it's intended to be irony – extremist Christian sects in North America condemn mothers for having tactile, and potentially sensual, contact with their children). Charlotte articulates the progressive point of view on the topic – that many cultures believe it's healthy for the baby, that it helps them to regulate their breathing (which falls into line with that of the mother, apparently). The downside is that you might roll over in your sleep and "squish" the baby in your sleep (the squishing is an urban myth, I think)...

Miranda ends up doubting herself. She feels she has no maternal instinct, no patience; she works 50 hours a week. She worries for the infant to-be...

Having been given some of the items she needs before she gets to the point when she can never leave her apartment again, Miranda (in *'I heart NY'*) asks Carrie to be at the birth with her. She doesn't want any cheerleader type stuff or anyone telling her to push; however, we never get to know the minutiae of her birth-plan (that's assuming she got around to writing one even after Charlotte's prompt). We only see the end of the labour and Miranda looks at Carrie and appears to have an orgasm (it was supposed to be an excruciatingly painful final contraction – ha, ha). Clearly, pain is something hard to enact, although there is a wacky American writer who apparently suggests that giving birth should be like having an orgasm. For those of us who had ***excruciatingly painful*** drug-free 'natural' home births, her name is mud. Perhaps the scriptwriters for *Sex and the City* had come across the concept?

The scene ends with Miranda having an emotional experience holding her baby – perhaps she does have maternal instinct after all? Yet, even in her tender mood, Miranda frowns at the progenitor, Steve, when it looks as if he's going to cry.

In *Friends,* baby Emma has disappeared entirely, leaving Rachael able to continue her character as before. Chandler and Monica go for fertility tests because they have been trying for over a year. Chandler doesn't want to 'deposit his specimen' in the container – he doesn't like the idea of undergoing these 'routine' tests. Just to make the scene in the clinic more excruciating, Chandler tries to joke with an unamused female medic and then runs into his ex-girlfriend, Janice. The episode ends with Chandler taking the call from the clinic with the results. They both have a problem: Monica has an inhospitable environment and Chandler's sperm have 'low motility' (that's sluggish sperm, and those that do make it are wiped out...).

Saturday 24th May 03.

Today I went out and bought newborn socks, little booties with a rattle in them, a newborn hat, mittens, newborn 'baby grow' and vest. I also bought a massive inflatable rattle (which was Emile's favourite toy for ages until he punctured it) all to send to my friend Becky... For Emile I bought crayons, cymbals, a triangle and castanets. I'd actually been looking for a new beater for his glockenspiel but will have to make a trip to a specialist music shop it seems. I also bought him a book with buttons which plays different tunes – he has a couple of these already and absolutely loves them. For Eilish I chose flashcards and she chose some cute T shirts. I didn't manage to buy anything for myself, though... We did make it into a woman's clothes shop, but at that precise moment Eilish announced that she needed the toilet...

Monday 26th May 03.

I've just spent the best part of two days in playgrounds (today's a bank holiday). Emile spent most of the afternoon pushing around his sister's dolly stroller and smiling benignly at the world (as well as flirtingly giving flowers to various women). Eilish did lots of vigorous climbing and high-speed sliding (sitting on her fleece to reduce the friction) and has mastered the monkey bars and figured out how to swing on her own – though she still likes to be pushed. Emile, on approaching the pond, said the word "duck". I feel quite bereft at the prospect of having to go back to work tomorrow.

Tuesday 27th May 03.

Our six year old, Eilish, is learning about adjectives at school so Robert chose six adjectives to describe the noun Eilish:

Cute
Sweet
Lovely
Delightful
Kind
Charming

For fun I did six too:

Loving
Sensitive
Imaginative
Playful
Kind
Clever

I think his were proscriptive and/or wishful thinking, whereas I think my adjectives more closely describe her personality. We agree she is kind.

Wednesday 28th May 03.
I just worked an eleven-hour day and then drove over an hour to get home. How did my life get so crazy? And what do I spend my wages on? – mortgages. Not only mortgages but mortgages on two empty houses. These are on the market but haven't sold. How did my life get so crazy?
On the way back, I was hoping Eilish would still be awake so I could read her a bedtime story. In fact, she was not only awake but dancing naked in the kitchen to loud Turkish pop music while Maristella cooked her a very late dinner (Robert, the routine keeper, is away). When she ate the strawberries I'd brought back with me, the juice dribbled down her tummy. She is a sensual little creature.
I've been told that no applications for part-time employment can be considered in my workplace for a year. Staff leaving are not being replaced. Consequently, heads of departments are not approving any applications from staff wishing to change from full-time to part-time contracts. I really don't know if I've got enough stamina to last another year full-time, emotionally or physically, and the idea of lecturing again through another pregnancy simply appals me.

Thursday 29th May 03.
Emile is 17 months old today and I took the day off work. Most of the time was spent in the park. He has become rather wilful. Once unleashed (for a ball game) he was unwilling to go back into his buggy. My attempts to get him strapped back resulted in a full tantrum with much writhing so I ended

up carrying him past the duck ponds and waterfalls to our destination. He played happily in a sand pit for over an hour and would have stayed longer except that Eilish had become restless. Once, at the main playground he mastered the slide and spent ages on the baby gym – tunnel, steps etc. It was a beautiful day, and apart from Eilish wading in the duck pond and getting her feet muddy, without incident. Why do I mention this? Well, because it is my enjoyment of my children that justifies the third. So I feel there is a link. Every time I really enjoy my children and give myself over to them fully I feel that perhaps it is not quite so insane to have another!

Friday 30th May 03.
In *Friends* Monica and Chandler are coming to terms with their fertility problems. She is amazed that she has an 'inhospitable environment' because she has always tried to be a good hostess and he is surprised that his sperm have 'low motility', as they have always seemed to be in a hurry to get places in the past. They discuss impregnation, sperm donorship and adoption.
There is a hilarious scene in which Chandler brings home an attractive male colleague and they grill him all evening about his health and heredity as a potential sperm donor (the guest not knowing what they have in mind but feeling increasingly nervous). When Monica says she doesn't want to have the other man's sperm Chandler retorts, "but he's better than me" – "sperm-tastic", in fact (Chandler's in advertising now). Monica only wants to have Chandler's baby. They end up resolving to explore adoption. Indeed what was striking, from a British perspective, was their smug certitude that a baby would be available for them…

Sunday 1st June 03.
I just read a very heart-rending piece in *The Guardian* Weekend by Emma Loach whose 20-week scan showed shadows on the foetus's heart. At first, she assumed the medic doing the scan was taking so long because he was young and inexperienced, but after an hour had passed I could palpably imagine her rising sense of panic. The measurements taken indicated Down's Syndrome. The article described what happened from there – waiting to see the Consultant the following week, her husband being utterly convinced that a mistake had been made, waiting for the

appointment whilst feeling the baby kicking vigorously – seemingly healthy, being scanned again and then being immediately referred for amniocentesis – the full results of which would not be ready, they were informed, for three long weeks. Then after three days came the call that confirmed that her 'baby' had Down's Syndrome and the piece described her and her partner's emotional breakdown on being told to come into the hospital immediately.

To terminate the pregnancy Emma had to take tablets and then return to the hospital three days later to give birth. This does seem inhumane to me – couldn't it be done in one day? She says of these few days that they were appalling:

> 'I felt like a murderer waiting to strike her victim. I used to think the feeling of your baby kicking inside you and the sight of the foot poking against your skin were the most fantastic things in the world. But for those few days they were torture. It felt as if we had gone power crazy. Elliot and I had so much power, we could decide that this little thing should die.'

The actual labour took 11 hours and then afterwards Emma had milk for weeks and of course there was the disposal of the little body. They had the corpse cremated. Now Emma is filled with feelings of self-loathing for killing her 'innocent unborn child'. The piece certainly brought home to me very vividly the horrendous, emotionally scarring cost of finding out so late that there is a serious problem.

Would I abort a seriously damaged foetus? Yes. I am forty-two so a chromosomal abnormality is a real possibility. Until I'd read Emma's article the full horrible implications of this hadn't sunk in; however, I shall have CVS at 10 or 11 weeks and if I am very 'lucky' the pregnancy could be over by the twelfth week so perhaps I might be spared the dreadful experience of feeling movement. Early terminations are less traumatic: the cervix is dilated and then the contents of the womb are sucked out. What Emma experienced is standard for very late terminations. The labour is induced, commonly with prostaglandin, and the woman goes into labour and 'gives birth' to a dead foetus.

Thursday 5th June 03.

I haven't been thinking about getting pregnant though it is constantly at the back of my mind. My latest period is just finishing. What did I experience when it arrived? I felt sad but there were no tears or emotional scenes this time. I'm coming to terms with the fact that it might take months or years or that it might never happen.

Thursday 12th June 03.

Last night I had a powerful dream in which I was in labour. Instead of feeling calm when I reached 'transition', the temporary calm before the enormous final contractions, I was struck by a terrible feeling of terror. Robert had gone out for something and I was about to give birth alone. I saw him approaching in the distance just before waking up…

Friday 13th June 03.

I keep forgetting to mention *Friends* in which baby Emma has entirely been dropped from the plot. In the last two episodes both parents, Rachael and Ross, have been at a palaeontology conference in Barbados at which Ross gave the keynote speech. Neither mentions the baby or makes anxious phone calls to Ross's mother (or whoever is supposed to be looking after her). Rachael, a few episodes ago, couldn't let baby Emma out of her sight – now it's a case of out of sight, out of mind.

Rachael is looking sexy again, after her brief maternal frumpy look, has been lusting after the hunky actor Joey and the episode closed with her having sex with Joey in her Barbados hotel room (or they appear to be about to have sex). Ross is about to have sex with a fellow palaeontologist. So both parents are having sex and enjoying their holiday in Barbados. I guess this should be welcomed – Rachael is not letting motherhood dominate her life, nor is she feeling obliged to try and make a go of it with Ross (to whom she seems immeasurably unsuited) just because they have had a baby together.

Saturday 14th June 03.

Tomorrow is father's day and Robert was complaining that the children make a mother's day card, but not a father's day card, at school. I was wondering what percentage of households actually has a resident father. It seems clear that the teachers are avoiding potential embarrassment to a number of pupils per class by not making the card.

The thought of absent fathers reminds me of a surprising news item reported in today's *Guardian*. Two 'unmarried' mothers were forced by a judges ruling (in a case brought against them by the children's 'fathers') to give their children the controversial MMR (measles, mumps and rubella) vaccine, a cocktail which has been linked to autism and dyslexia. (I'd be interested to know if the drug companies funded the court case?). Why I found this ruling surprising was that the mothers are looking after the children. Therefore, if the vaccine disables the children it will be the mothers (not the fathers) who have to deal with the consequences. Likewise, if their children contracted measles, they'd also be doing the care. I thought this an extraordinary imposition on the judge's part. (Yes, I am fully aware of arguments about 'herd immunity' but think them irrelevant in this case).

Furthermore, the fathers were not reported as being 'unmarried', though clearly they were not married to the women in question. The term 'unmarried mothers' carries with it a whiff of judgement I thought, and why talk about the marital status of the mothers but not the fathers? The ruling considerably undermines the woman's parental authority. Moreover, it is likely that the situation was extremely acrimonious for the men to behave in this way, and the atmosphere for the children will hardly be improved by the outcome – the judge should have supported the women's decision. That a man who is not the husband and who is not resident with the children should be able to exert this kind of influence over day to day parenting decisions is extremely worrying. I chose to give MMR to both my children (though with misgivings) but it is outrageous that mothers should not have the right to choose on this issue. Women should be able to mother their children without undue interference from ex-partners or sperm donors.

In the afternoon I took both children to the local park and I felt utterly contented though I have to admit I did once, fleetingly, imagine myself with three children. Someone I know (but who didn't know I had children) greeted us as we were on the cycle path, Emile in his buggy and Eilish sitting on the front having a ride (fortunately, I have what may be the most robust buggy on the market). She made the kind of remark that people make, "you've got your hands full", or some such thing. It was then that I imagined a new born baby strapped to my front. Am I buying into the superwoman thing? We were walking too slowly for my acquaintance to walk with us for long and once Emile was unleashed from his buggy I really did have my hands full. We did manage a tranquil half-an-hour under a big tree at one point. Emile sat or pottered about drinking his juice while Eilish made a sculpture of Rapunzel out of newly cut grass and decorated her hair with twigs and flowers.

Sunday15th June 03.

Today is day 14 of my cycle so I could be ovulating. I started using the douche again a couple of days ago. I was feeling very sensual this morning wrapped around Robert's chunky, hairy, little body in bed, but he's not very keen on morning sex, generally. This is my favourite time of day for love making so I am disappointed by his recent lack of interest when we have the opportunity (which is rarely because of children needing to be looked after). This morning he was a bit hung-over so not to be tempted. Actually, I love daytime sex. I like to stand and look at the person I'm making love to and peel their clothes off very very slowly… I can feel very sensual in the afternoons around ovulation time. Maristella has just taken both children to a multi-cultural festival so Robert and I are alone together in the house, which is rare. We could be at it like rabbits but Robert is not often keen on daytime sex. Besides, he is engrossed in *The Observer* and therefore unlikely to be amenable to anything until he is sated.

Our problem is that Emile never goes to bed before 9.00pm so early evening sex is out, and besides, Robert doesn't feel sexy when he's around the baby. So long as the baby was engrossed in something, as he sometimes is, I wouldn't have a problem having sex while Emile was with us, but since Robert does have a problem with it my willingness is irrelevant. Depending on when I got up and what I've been doing I can be quite tired by 9.30pm, so while I'm still definitely 'up for' sex, as the expression goes, I can be slightly off-peak by the time we get around to it. Anyway, tonight is definitely going to include sex because I may be ovulating.

I realise, writing this, that I am feeling quite sexually frustrated. Around my ovulation I just want sex all the time and we haven't had sex since Friday night, which feels like an age ago!

Monday 16th June 03.

I asked a group of my post-graduate students what they thought about the recent MMR controversy. They were either undecided or thought the judge's decision wrong. Two of them revealed, coincidentally, that they were working for advocacy groups for fathers, and an interesting discussion ensued. One was working for an organisation, the name of which I won't reveal, with a policy to not work with men who had been violent or who are drug addicts (she used the term 'substance abusers' which perhaps includes alcoholism); however, she revealed, very interestingly, that in confidential group work, "the majority of the men revealed that they had been violent" at some point, either towards their ex-partners or to their children.

It was only afterwards that I wondered about the ethics of such organisations negotiating custody and access orders for violent men who are obviously plausible liars. No wonder the women "often didn't co-operate" – they know their ex is a violent, lying bastard. Personally, I wouldn't want a man who'd smashed me in the face anywhere near my children, or me **ever again**. That his sperm was involved in their creation seems frankly irrelevant.

Tuesday 17th June 03.

More sex with Robert in case my ovulation is late. I've been feeling shattered so wonder if I am pregnant already? It might just be my age though…

Wednesday 18th June 03.

Maristella has been in a black mood all day because I had words with her about her lack of punctuality and tendency to disappear at times when she is supposed to be working. Sometimes it feels to me that someone is always in a strop in this house.

Thursday 19th June 03.

I hope Emile won't end up having an identity crisis as a consequence of the remarkable number of nicknames he has. A few have fallen into disuse. An early one, 'Plumpington' sounds to me a bit like a Victorian storybook character: Mr Plumpington surveyed his surroundings… But we don't want Emile to be worried about his plumpness so we stopped using it. At the moment, Robert calls him: 'tuppy' and 'tuppy moo-moo'. Indeed, "I want to bite into your plump, juicy moo-moos" is a frequent refrain in this house. Fortunately, he's too young to realise how mad we all are. Other of Robert's favourites are: 'tuppy-hoga', 'tup tup', 'plooper', 'proud peacock', 'chupatoos' and 'vous maj'. His six year old sister has come up with: 'Emilio', 'Emilkio', 'drinkio', and 'chuppy' (as a corruption of cubby). I call him 'babaganoosh', 'tuppy', 'tuppiness' or just 'baba'. I even call him Emile. Our au-pair, Maristella, calls him 'Mr Majesty'.

Friday 20th June 03.

I've been living with Robert for six months today. Peculiar how it feels as though I've always been living with him…

Saturday 21st June 03.

Today Eilish left two bits of lettuce and some red pepper, walnut and pomegranate paté on her plate after lunch and because I didn't make her eat it Robert sulked for about two hours for "undermining him". He didn't even tell her to eat it. Not actively backing his regime without being asked to do so can't properly be said to be 'undermining', in my view. Furthermore, I'm supposed to do it though I don't actually agree with making people eat things they don't want to eat. She looked so miserable at the prospect I let her off. I think Robert's being over ambitious in what he expects a six year old to eat and ridiculous in behaving as though it's a big deal… As I said, someone is always in a strop in this house.

Monday 23rd June 03.

A number of my students know that my recent research has been on support for women who are pregnant or have recently given birth. I got interested in this subject after having had quite a traumatic first labour.

Over coffee, and quite without prompting, one of my students revealed that he had had a vasectomy because the birth of his child had been so distressing. It was a long and painful labour resulting in an episiotomy, the use of forceps and ventouse (a suction cap which is inserted into the virgina and attached to the baby's scalp – once enough suction has been achieved the baby is pulled out). He said that he never wanted his wife to go through that again.

Tuesday 24th June 03.
I've been reading Sylvia Hewlett's *Baby Hunger*, which I've found absolutely riveting. It's about how high-achieving women don't have children and then regret it. I actually meet her definition of a high-achieving woman, by salary (I scrape in at the bottom) and professional status (I'm a University Reader at time of writing, soon to be a Professor, perhaps…), so am quite enthralled by some of her research findings.
For example, in her sample of women aged 41-55, **only 1%** had given birth to a first child after the age of thirty-nine. **None of the women with salaries over $100,000 had had a first child over the age of 36.**
Why don't high achieving women have babies? According to Hewlett, women often put off finding a partner and having children until it's too late and their fertility is declining. In their thirties many high-achieving women are prioritising their careers. Then, when these women want to find a partner, they discover that their male colleagues are either already married or simply not interested. Hewlett suggests that high achieving women want to be with successful men but that successful men want, generally, to be with less ambitious women who work shorter hours and are consequently more available (this is based on America where executives work longer hours than in Europe). The men are looking for someone who will complement them rather than someone who is experiencing similar pressures and stresses and working crazy hours.
Why high-powered women don't turn to, what Australians call SNAGS, (sensitive new age guys), isn't explored. There must be quite a few unambitious men or struggling writers or artists who'd be happy to be kept, and to keep house, in America? (Incidentally, when I worked in Australia, I had a cartoon on my office door with a picture of some macho Australian men having a barbecue ('barbie') in the outback. The text read,

“toss another SNAG on the Barbie, Bruce”). Anyway, I feel sympathetic to SNAGS.

Successful women are happier continuing to engage in some work, than quitting altogether, when they do manage to have children. Hewitt’s basic argument is that staff turnover actually costs many businesses more (in readvertising, recruitment and retraining) than it would to introduce ‘work-life’ balance policies such as, fractional posts, flexi-time, parenting leave, and so on, to encourage women to stay on after they have children. She is very persuasive, so much so, that she is listened to be government ministers and corporate chiefs.

Wednesday 25th June 03.

My friend Becky left a text message on my phone saying she is going through hell. When I phoned her, she said that she wished that she’d never got pregnant – and this is someone who once described her *raison d’etre* as having children. With rocketing blood pressure, she had spent two nights in the hospital this week. At one point, she was told that she should consider having an emergency Caesarean but she challenged the evidence put before her. I made the point that at least as an assertive and intelligent person she couldn’t be completely intimidated but that’s not how she feels. She said she feels completely “taken over” and that there is “nothing” of her left… She said that dealing with the NHS is a “nightmare”, that she is constantly referred from one person to another, that the decisions taken are poor, that scans have been misread. She is on a “cocktail” of drugs and her blood pressure keeps rising to such an extent that she in danger of having a stroke. Furthermore, she has been described as “aggressive” in her notes. She is exhausted and scared.

The most outrageous thing that happened is that, on one occasion having had no sleep at the hospital, she decided to discharge herself, on so doing she refused the offer of a further scan. The nurse on duty retorted, “you’ll be coming back with a dead baby inside you”.

I suggested that she see an independent midwife but she seems to be utterly convinced that she can’t have a normal birth and is considering having an elective Caesarean at 38 weeks (she is 34 weeks at present).

Thursday 26th June 03.
Becky texted me this morning to say that her blood pressure has shot up and she may be having an emergency Caesarean. I am feeling nervous and can't relax because she may be on the operating table as I write.

Friday 27th June 03.
I've just been reading the section on in vitro fertilisation in Sylvia Hewlett's *Baby Hunger.* I don't think British women have the same expectations of late in life pregnancies, as the American women she quotes. The statistics are sobering. By the age of thirty-nine the success rate of IVF is only 8% and by the time women are forty-four the success rate has fallen to only 3%, and it's very, very expensive and may have cancer risks attached to it.
What exactly is IVF? Drugs are taken to stimulate the production of eggs (the side effects of these are not very nice). Then before ovulation occurs a fine probe, guided by an ultrasound, is inserted into the ovary through the vaginal wall (ouch). The eggs, which have been monitored for their maturity, are placed in an incubator with the sperm for fertilisation to take place. These are then inserted into the uterus. Two weeks later a pregnancy test can be taken to see if the procedure has been successful. Because embryos can be destroyed in this process, some extremist Christian sects have always been opposed to it.
Reading this book had made me realise that my blithe assumption that I can definitely have a third baby might be wrong. This idea has was emphasised by the fact that that my period has started. No trauma this time as I'm getting used to thinking that this could take a while.

Saturday 28th June 03.
This morning I found a text from Becky on my mobile confirming that she is out of hospital and has not had a Caesarean. I don't want to intrude too much as I know, from talking to other women, that all the "have you had the baby yet?" phone calls can become rather wearing.
I was performing today. I sing in a world music group (one of my last remaining hobbies not to have been obliterated by motherhood). I took Eilish along to watch and join in. Until I moved to Sheffield, I always used to take her with me to choir practice but the choir I now sing with meets

quite late and isn't overtly 'child-friendly'. She was very well behaved and joined in when we did some audience participation; however, what really excited her was the Indian henna hand painting and my buying her some Indian bracelets. Six year olds are so easy to please…

Sunday 29th June 03.
Emile was one-and-a-half today so we had a cake with one-and-a-half candles. This was mainly for Eilish's amusement of course, but he did manage to blow them out.

Tuesday 1st July 03.
I've just spent 17 hours in the office in the last two days (normally I spend at least eighteen to twenty plus hours in the office from Monday morning to returning to Sheffield on Tuesday evening (– not including the commuting time – add that and I've done about 22 hours. Then I do a minimum of one hour, work related, reading after the children have gone to bed – making a total of at least 24 hours). Most of it was spent in meetings putting in, what Hewlett calls, 'face time'. None of the meetings I attended really required my attendance. The managers of particular courses could give the course and module reports – there is absolutely no need for all teaching staff to be there. Furthermore, I did not learn any crucial information which will enable me to improve my performance in the forthcoming academic year. This is corporate culture infiltrating universities. I am seen to be part of the team. I would rather be getting on with some research or teaching preparation or even administration. But I sit and sit pointlessly. If I were going to sit doing nothing, I'd rather be doing it watching my lovely eighteen-month old son pottering around. Indeed, he is very busy. When I'm with him in the garden he never stops. He shovels up a spade of sand and carries it to some other point in the garden. He moves toys around. He picks a flower and hands it to me. He climbs into his toy car and out again and continues like this for hours, almost without respite. All the activity is fundamentally pointless. And I think most of my work time is just the same, except that what I do is much much more complex.

Friday 4th July 03.

I read this headline today: 'Each year an estimated 530,000 women die during pregnancy or childbirth. Most deaths occur in developing countries and most are preventable'. It was an advertisement for staff to work on researching maternal mortality so it didn't say what was causing all these deaths. Post-partum infections a lot of them, I guess. I feel I should know more about this.

Saturday 5th July 03.

Following a sudden and intense burst of discontent, for the first time in the seven years I'm job hunting. I've applied for five jobs in the last few days and I've already been short-listed for one. It feels bizarre to be applying for jobs when in a few days time I could be pregnant again. Robert says I should apply because I might not become pregnant or it that it might take years for me to become pregnant. I feel that it's bizarre that I might be sitting, already pregnant, in a job interview next Friday. My ovulation will occur sometime between Thursday and Sunday and of course we'll be having Wednesday evening sex before I go to London (I'll sleep in a hotel because it's an all-day interview).

Sunday 6th July 03.

Robert unveiled Eilish's end of year report over dinner. To my surprise, because she was defined as having `special needs' at her last school, she got in the 22 subject areas, 17 `excellent' scores and 5 'very good' scores (and nothing else). Robert read them out one by one in quite a dramatic performance. (There are times when I feel intense love for Robert, and that was one of them). Maristella has given her the nickname "excellent Eilish" which should help to boost her academic confidence. It just goes to show how children have developmental spurts and can more than catch up when lagging behind – though it's a shame that so much attention is focused on developmental norms rather than an acceptance of difference. I felt so sorry for Eilish when she started to become embarrassed that her reading ability was not as good as some of the others in the class. Briefly last year, she even developed a hostile aversion to trying to read; however, because her time with mummy is so valued as soon I took over the reading and homework from Delphine (who had terrific English) she began to

regain her enthusiasm. We are a bookish family. She will see Robert and I reading every day and she knows that "mummy writes books".
This reminds me of the terrible problems my friend Michelle is having trying to get her local secondary school, at which Jasmine is about to start in September, to implement their policy of 'social inclusion'. So, for example, Jasmine, who wears leg splints and sometimes uses a wheelchair too, has been put in a class that has its registration on the top floor of the building (there is no lift). She has quite severe 'learning difficulties' but the use of certain aids, such as a recording machine (for messages from the home to the school about what Jasmine has been doing and vice-versa) has been deemed "inappropriate". Furthermore, she has not been put in the same class as her best friend. These are just a few of the problems. Additionally, in attempting to address this fiasco, my friend has met with a hostile and defensive response. My life is easy in comparison.

Wednesday 9th July 03.
I had quite a long conversation with Becky's mother-in-law who answered the phone when I rang. Becky has had an emergency Caesarean and is feeling quite ill and rather miserable. The baby was only a little over three pounds but seems quite normal and is in an incubator. I sent the congratulations card I had ready. I think it's cruel the way people in hospital are prevented from using their mobile phones and are consequently isolated from their friends and family.

Thursday 10th July 03.
All week I've been traumatised over whether or not to attend the job interview tomorrow. I phoned this morning to say I was withdrawing my application. If I'm pregnant, the last thing I need is a long commute and two nights away from my family each week. It's more money, and potentially better terms and conditions – I should say 'was'. I can't phone back and say I've changed my mind and will attend the interview after all! Significantly, they were willing to offer a good working at home agreement.
I was actually in tears this morning and I've managed to do no research all week because I've been so preoccupied with the interview and writing the presentation I was to give. I woke up this morning and thought – I can't

go! It's been a waste of a week of annual leave apart from my jaunt into London with Eilish on Monday and Tuesday, which was fun (we watched some fascinating footage of eggs moving down fallopian tubes and cells dividing to become a foetus following fertilisation, at the Natural History Museum). We stayed with a friend of mine who has a 50K local government job and is a single parent with THREE children. That she keeps it all together (even with a little help from dope and amphetamines) is nothing short of miraculous. Her house is immaculately tidy (except the children's rooms, of course); however, Robert sulked and was angry for two days on my return because we looked up my ex-mother-in-law. He only calmed down again late last night. I never promised to cut off my ex in-laws when we got together. He is being very unreasonable and a bully. I have never met anyone less willing to compromise.

Friday 11th July 03.

Having pulled out of the interview I suddenly felt very calm and as I sat in the garden with my toddler I thought how I'd rather be doing that than strutting about in a power suit. (The job was a Head of Department's job and the directorship of a research institute). Perhaps I'll be disappointed, but I want to have the time to go to the local mother and baby group. I want to have much more time to just be with my children – I think a reduced hours contract may be the answer. When I think about any given week, the highlights are almost always the moments I manage to spend with the children.

I could be ovulating today so Robert and I made a point of having an early night. We had sex last night, too.

Saturday 12th July 03.

I came across a very interesting article which said that a leading health insurer was no longer willing to pay for 'convenience Caesareans' The insurer 'has said that it will no longer pay for Caesarean births because of uncertainty over whether the procedure is medically necessary.' That sounds like good news to me, as it's a very dangerous procedure, with all kinds of complications attached to it, which tend not to be explained. It's very overused, according to the article; over 50% of all births in some private hospitals are now by Caesarean. I can understand women wanting to avoid the pain of labour (they should realise that Caesareans are painful afterwards) but one thing we can be absolutely sure of is that women have always endured it.

Tuesday 15th July 03.
I finally remembered to ask the swimming pool attendant about the PH level of the pool. It's slightly alkaline rather than PH neutral (giving the advantage to male sperm). I didn't swim until day 16 this cycle but if I ovulated late that might have had a crucial impact. Well, if I'm not pregnant this month I'll definitely not swim anywhere near my ovulation time again (I really want a girl).

Thursday 17th July 03.
It's interesting how trying to get pregnant has distorted our sex. Robert now wants to save himself for my fertile period, although I've tried to persuade him that having more sperm wont make conception much more likely. He's very lacking in stamina for such a young person. I should have picked someone twenty years younger, rather than a mere decade younger! Anyway, I just mention this because after our Sunday sex (in case of late ovulation) there hasn't been any… He gives me cunnilingus to stop me going mad.

Friday 18th July 03
Robert told me he read an article today in a newspaper which said that women were more likely to have subsequent miscarriages if their first child had been a boy. He couldn't recall the details – frustratingly.

Saturday 19th July 03.
Robert was deliberately unkind and aggressive this evening. I ended up weeping with a depth of feeling and ferocity I had not experienced for a while. When was the last time I cried like that? Then I remembered, it was when I was about one week pregnant. It's something to do with the dramatic change in hormones, I suppose. During my last two pregnancies, just a few days after conception, I experienced a cathartic release of emotions (there was a trigger in both instances – but my depth of feeling was particularly strong). I'm not going to say anything to Robert, because

I know he'll be gutted if I have got this wrong. I think I am pregnant. Sometimes, 'older' women like me conceive and then miscarry almost immediately, so until my period is at least a week late I'll not do a test. As someone who has been pregnant three times, I should know how soon a result can be obtained, but I don't. I've always ***known***, so have never rushed out early for a pregnancy test. I should start feeling ill pretty soon if I am pregnant. The first ten weeks is like having a bad virus for me. For other women it's different. Some feel absolutely wonderful and extra libidinous; others can't keep food down or lead normal lives. With Emile, I lost the capacity to have orgasms after 22 weeks which was rather disappointing because when I was pregnant with Eilish I'm sure I experienced heightened sexual feelings for longer than that, but had no sexual partner.

Sunday 20th July 03.
Emile bit Eilish today. It was quite a nasty bite. Ever since Emile has been capable of holding objects Eilish has abruptly snatched the object of his interest – not a nice habit. He squeals vigorously when it happens and is sometimes so enraged that he will lash out at whoever is closest – including me.

The Observer had quite an interesting piece, melodramatically entitled *'War Zone NHS drives women to home births'*, on women who are so terrified of interference they have their children at home with no midwife present – misleadingly, these are called 'unattended births'. One woman was told that she had a potentially fatal condition which would require a hospital birth. She was determined to have a home birth. She did. She set up a birth pool in her kitchen and gave birth with her husband and son for company. The really audacious thing about 'Laura' was that she then "wrapped a big towelling robe around the two of us and went to bed".
You have a healthy baby and you are exhausted, of course the rational thing to do is to go to bed and sleep as Laura did; however, the socially acceptable thing to do is to phone the midwifery team, lie (if you don't want a confrontation) that it happened very quickly and then allow them to intrude on your privacy. They will satisfy themselves that the baby is breathing normally, will weigh and measure the baby (which will probably

make it cry, perhaps for the first time) inspect your virgina and perineum for tearing (not nice if you are feeling tender), pressurise you into taking drugs if you have not already delivered the placenta and so on… In other words, they will generally make a nuisance of themselves at a moment which may, or may not, have been beautiful and intimate.
Laura's local health authority responded to her decision to flout social convention (though her behaviour is probably indicative of centuries of practice of letting the mother follow her intuition about the birth) by attempting to have the baby removed into care on the grounds that Laura had put the two of them at risk. Fortunately, the local authority was unsuccessful in having the baby removed. Personally, I'd like to slap the person in the health authority who tried to take that line.
Laura's case has just been presented to the House of Commons Select Committee on Health, which is on the verge of making a pronouncement about birthing services. Health Secretary, John Reid, is intending to extend patient choice in maternity services – whatever that means.

Monday 21st July 03.
I turned on the radio and heard the term 'foeticide' for the first time and was transfixed. The programme was about sex selection through the selective abortion of foetuses; however, it is female foetuses that are being selected because of the high value placed on sons in Indian society as well as the costs associated with dowries for daughters. This is a practice so widespread in parts of Southern India that it has significantly skewed the normal ratio of girls to boys.
A few years ago, told the report, advertising used to promote the practice of aborting female foetuses in a highly public manner, with huge billboard posters promoting the idea with slogans such as 'spend 5 rupees today' (the cost of the ultra-sound examination) 'and save 500,000 rupees later'… (the cost of the bride's dowry at her marriage).
The use of ultra-sound to determine the sex for purposes of sex selection is now illegal in India but the practice is still rife.
The rest of the programme was about the murder of brides whose fathers don't cough-up enough cash. What has been termed 'dowry murders' are still a daily occurrence.

Tuesday 22nd July 03.
I am feeling rather queasy still. This could be it.

Wednesday 23th July 03.
My period is due tomorrow. This is the moment of truth. I think I am pregnant and that there will be no period this month.

Thursday 24th July 03.
My period started last night. I'm developing a bad cold, so that's why I was feeling ill. I feel nothing at all. No, that's not true. I feel mild relief that the drama, which I feel sure will happen at some point, is not happening right now. Emile has been waking in the night. Sometimes he just lies in his cot and burbles or sings. Frequently, he goes back to sleep without either of us having to get up. His noise wakes me up though. Robert has been waking very early. He wakes me up too. The idea of night-feeding a new born baby on top of this is hard to imagine, though at least I'd get a decent maternity leave this time because of the new EC legislation, so I'd be able to nap during the day to make up for the deficit. With Emile I had only three short months before I had to return to my job, which is not long enough to recover ones energy and after a few months back in the fray I was feeling absolutely exhausted. I'll definitely take the maximum maternity leave next time – assuming there is a next time.

Saturday 2nd Aug 03.
Robert and I have been staying at a resort in Tunisia that I visited before, two years ago, with Eilish (in the days before I moved in with Robert and can no longer take holidays as I please). Although I was having a harmonious and enjoyable time with Robert and really enjoying his company (perhaps more than ever before), I realised mid-way though that I really wanted Eilish to be there.
All the time, I was reminded of the things we'd done together two years ago and I found myself missing her constantly (though I could also recall some low points of the holiday, especially her refusal to dress for dinner one night and my marching her up to the restaurant almost naked, me fuming and carrying her clothes in a plastic bag, and then making her dress at the restaurant door). It's the first time I realise I really resent

Robert preventing my having a holiday with her, I'll have to try to negotiate that she and I have a special holiday together in future.
It's hard adjusting to being in a family after having been a single parent when I could do as I pleased. Robert constantly cuts across my wishes and desires.

Sunday 3rd Aug 03.
This is the last day of our holiday and possibly my first fertile day (day 12) so we had morning sex before our flight. It has to be said that Robert is always able to perform when required. He is clearly very keen to have a baby. It's just as well our holiday isn't longer as he's got to the stage when he's doing baby talk with other peoples babies (our children are with his parents in Stevenage). He'll start embracing other people's kids soon, so good to get him home.

Monday 4th Aug 03.
At lunch with Robert's parents and Maristella, Eilish wasn't very hungry and asked for "pudding" before we'd finished the main course. She responded well to being asked to wait but, knowing it was the last day of the holiday, asked for a second pudding after the first (we only have fresh fruit at home). She wanted jelly. Meanwhile, Emile was busy throwing his food on the floor… There was the usual tension between Robert's parents: Jacquie and Rumy. I thought it quite a successful lunch, but Robert fell into a foul mood because of Eilish's "brattish behaviour". He went off and read the newspaper and watched the news for two hours while I played with the children in the garden. This irked me as he said he'd missed them; however, I though it better to give him the opportunity to regain his good humour so I left him alone. He didn't. Later on, confronting him, I asserted that I hadn't seen any "brattish behaviour" but I had noticed his bad mood… etc. Robert remained in a bad mood all day and I ended up telling him he was a "prat".

Tuesday & Wednesday 5/6th Aug 03.
I'm back in the office and working long days. There just seems to me an extraordinary amount of administration. Because I work late I sleep overnight near my office, I always find the silence and space quite strange

when I'm cut off from my family… Unfortunately, I'm usually too tired, having worked a ten plus hour day in the office, to use the time in a constructive way. I do manage my only regular long bath.

Thursday 7th Aug 03.

I've just read a chapter on death and dying in childbirth. It's research for the book I'm working on. It's certainly dispelled any romantic notions I might have had about 'natural' midwife supported childbirth in the good old days before modern male dominated obstetric interventions (though doctors did cause fatal infections by using unsterile forceps). It's clear that midwifery practices varied a great deal across Europe in the 18th and 19th Centuries, along with varied levels or training and competence, and that consequently maternal and child mortality varied because of these practices. Furthermore, the mortality rates were probably much higher than had previously been thought because bacterial infections resulting in, for example, Gastric Fever, were not realised to be related to infection at birth.

Friday - Saturday 8 - 11th August 03.

I'm back into the throng. The last few days have been busy including my trying to teach Eilish to swim in a local pool and visits to the Hillsborough Leisure Centre where both children like bobbing about in the machine generated waves or squirted with great jets of water. We've got lots of books from the library for Eilish. Robert's doing a daily maths and English session with her. She's doing art at the kitchen table right now. We've even had a family outing to the park – a rare occurrence, as Robert's a bit agoraphobic!

I'm now on holiday for the rest of the month, though I'm sure the time will disappear in flash. If this morning is anything to go by, it will.

Whilst sitting here, I've just been interrupted by Emile wandering in three times (he likes running about from room to room at the moment). Eilish wanted me to see a drawing she's working on and I have been summoned twice to appreciate it. Maristella had been in and Robert accounts for about eight other interruptions (wanting me to help him put the duvet in its cover and admire the newly tidied linen cupboard, amongst others). At one point, our for sale board was delivered and planted in the front garden

(I should say 'his' for sale board) so the entire family came in to watch this momentous occasion from this room, which gives the best view to the proceedings. I'm amazed I ever get any writing done at all. Now Robert wants me to do something regarding the joint account we've just opened so I'm going to give this up for today!

Saturday 16th Aug 03.

My favourite soap, *Sex in the City*, isn't focussing on Miranda's pregnancy. There were a few interesting scenes following the birth of Miranda's baby, one when the girls eye the baby suspiciously over brunch and Miranda tells them just to regard it like a big handbag! (They seem relived that nothing is expected of them, though Samantha, the least maternal, is positively dying to get rid of mother and babe so she can focus on some serious shopping – or perhaps she thinks having a baby in tow will put men off from flirting with her – her *raison d'etre*). There was a terrifically funny scene shortly after the birth in which Carrie could not concentrate on what Miranda was telling her because she couldn't take her eyes off Miranda's hugely engorged throbbing, veined breast, exposed while she breast feeds. The lack of empathy between those who don't have children – called 'child-free' in the USA – and those that do might have been further explored. The issue was touched upon when Samantha baby-sits Brady so that Miranda can attend a hairdressing appointment. When the electric rocking machine breaks down and the baby screams – Samantha, who is incapable of cuddling a baby, finds out that her newly bought vibrator has a soothing effect as the baby cuddles it!

Now the focus of attention is more on the relationship between Miranda and Steve (the baby's progenitor). They are not in a relationship, except that of co-parenting. In *To Market, To Market,* Miranda decides that she is in love with Steve. She invites him to dinner to tell him. Steve, assuming she is going to tell him to back off further, pre-empts her disclosure by announcing that she shouldn't worry because he is no longer in love with her and is seeing someone. Miranda is gutted and bemoans her status as a 37-year-old single mother – which is precisely what she wanted to be in the first place – man free.

Sex and the City does try for iconoclasm, and I hadn't seen a mother smear her brow accidentally with shit before on screen, whilst distractedly changing a nappy. It reminds me of my waving Robert, in his pin stripe suit, off to work from my house in Derby and noticing, just as he was about to leave, that one of the sleeves of his jacket was covered in baby shit. He was mortified about the fact that he might have turned up for work thus attired! Anyway, Miranda does manage to smear shit on herself (Steve is teasing her whilst holding the baby and trying to wipe the shit off with a baby wipe in a playful way) and this is the moment of her epiphany; she would like them to be a family.

Miranda is being depicted increasingly as a rather pathetic figure (though she has had one brief fling since having the baby) obsessed with watching television and eating chocolate cake. We don't get to see her enjoy the baby (she tends to pick Brady up when he's crying). Having a baby is depicted as a chore. In the following episode, *'The Perfect Present'*, over brunch with the girls, she finds a roll of Steve's condoms in the baby's nappy bag which the baby grabs and puts in his mouth. Miranda's look of alarm prompts Samantha's wonderful line, "Oh honey relax, I have those in my mouth all the time". When Steve arrives (late) to collect the baby, Miranda confronts him about the condoms, accuses him of not taking parenthood seriously and explodes into a fit of unseemly jealously (so distracted are they that the baby falls off the sofa).

Tuesday 19th Aug 03.

Today is day 28 of my cycle and no period. I am feeling nervous. I'm also feeling very tired. This could be because:

I'm aging

I'm on holiday and therefore relaxing, which is tiring

I ate too much for lunch and it's two-thirty in the afternoon (my sleepy patch in the day)

I never get a decent night's sleep anymore because of Robert's nightly thrashings about in bed or the baby waking.

I'm excited (which is tiring) about our offer on our *new house* being accepted and nervous (which is also tiring) that we might be gazumped

I'm naturally enervated before each period, but hadn't noticed prior to this attempt at trying to get pregnant

I am finally pregnant after seven months of trying.

Wednesday 20th Aug 03.
The estate agent's financial advisor rang up while I was out and Robert mentioned that this place (his house, in which we all currently reside) is on the market (which it hadn't been earlier). Then we both received messages on our mobiles saying, "this was not the basis on which the offer was accepted" (this presumably being a knee-jerk response to the dread of 'chains'). I've phoned the agent twice and not got hold of her. I left a message saying that the purchase is not dependant on the sale of this house (which is true as I've received a cash offer on my cottage in Derbyshire). I'll be gutted if we don't get this house. I've even told Eilish (who viewed the property with me) which room will be her bedroom!
And my period came again, as it seems to do with monotonous regularity. At least we got the mobile messages after I'd had a lovely morning in the park with the children. I've certainly been feeling wretched all afternoon!

Thursday 21st Aug 03.
I remind myself that I must remain 'in the here and now'. I mustn't waste my energy obsessing over a baby I don't have and might never have.

Friday 22nd Aug 03.
Emile had his late MMR and didn't even cry. He just looked puzzled as the nurse stuck the syringe in.

Saturday & Sunday 23-24th Aug 03.
Robert took Emile to London and he has been quite a handful. He didn't want to sleep at his normal time on the train and screamed for over five minutes. Robert was mortified. When Emile was put to bed at his normal time, after finishing his bottle he got up, opened the bedroom door, ran along a long corridor (which has a steep staircase) and into the lounge where he continued to demand lively attention. Vicci, (Robert's friend's fiancée) eventually took him to bed and stayed stroking him until he fell asleep. The following day he managed several spectacular tantrums when he didn't get his own way. Robert was very relieved to hand him over to me on his return.

Monday 25th Aug 03.
My friend Becky, who is now at home with her first baby, told me that she is never going to have another. I felt that this was a shame as perhaps a second pregnancy could be managed differently, but, of course, I wasn't the one with blood pressure so high I might have died; I have not endured a Caesarean Section either.

Thursday 28th Aug 03.
There have been no entries in this diary for the past few days because our au-pair has been away on holiday and we have been 'viewing' this house, as the expression goes…, 'exhibiting' the house would be more apt. We have had a steady stream of people through the place, even unexpected evening viewers (who the agent forgot to tell us about), so we have been on view whilst eating and also while the kids were having their bath – Eilish immediately struck a cute, I'm about to be photographed, pose. So, I've not had not much time to sit at my P.C.. We got the survey report on our new house through too and that looks good. The new house is huge – it will be wonderful to have room to move about…

Friday 29th Aug 03.
Today I spent the day at the Yorkshire Sculpture Park with my children and a friend and her thirteen-year-old son. Eilish ran around wildly with 'Neo' whilst Emile (who has been a bit unhappy since his MMR) caressed Barbara Hepworth sculptures, waddled around, and was generally a rather subdued. Emile is twenty months old today. I joked with passers by that you can never start their aesthetic appreciation too early. This is the last day of our summer holiday. I can't believe I'm due back at work next week.

Saturday 30th Aug 03.
Day twelve of my cycle so sex is guaranteed tonight. That's one of the good things about this 'trying for a baby' thing. There's no wondering if he'll be too tired or in the right mood. He's all ready and waiting with a massive erection.
Talking of massive erections, I asked Robert – if there were one thing he could change about his body – what would it be. I was assuming he'd say

he'd like to be a bit taller (he's only my height). He replied that he'd like a "massive dick". Even after I asserted that penetrative sex would be uncomfortable if he were a lot bigger – he still said he'd have to have a bigger dick! This is clearly nothing to do with his capacity to pleasure me. This is a male competitive thing. Evidently, he has been listening to too much hip-hop which has lyrics such as "put your tongue on my python" and "give it to me in your mouth" – not exact quotes to avoid having to request copyright clearance – but you get the picture…

Sunday 31th Aug 03.

Last night I forgot to use my vinegar solution douche (to preference 'female' sperm) and it's made me wonder if I'm feeling more relaxed about the possibility of having another boy. My swimming is slightly boy preferencing (the pool water being alkaline) and I'm due to swim later today too with the children… Today is day thirteen, more sex to follow.

This weekend's *Guardian* had a debate between a journalist and head of *Care* (an IVF provider). It was sparked off by the proposal from the National Institute for Clinical Excellence (Nice) that all infertile couples should receive NHS support for three cycles of fertility treatment – never mind that it fails three quarters of the time, that it's heinously expensive, invasive, that it may be associated with cancer (the cancer risk wasn't mentioned by either journalist or doctor). Dr Simon Fichel suggested that an equitable policy on infertility treatment was long overdue. He also stated that good IVF practice can offer a 1:3 chance of conception, hence 'we are now doing better than nature.'

Fichel gets lyrical, suggesting that 'fertility transcends culture, nationhood, religion… consider', he continues, 'if mankind awoke tomorrow to find not a single fertile individual on the planet – then where would be the hope, the future, the meaning to life?' Given that about half of all British women now opt not to have children (or have fertility problems which prevent them having children) it seems that a lot of people really don't care much about the continuance of the species – and it doesn't stop them appearing to be quite happy.

Anyway, this is something of a digression, as middle ground was found between the two in thinking the industry funded regulatory body (the human fertilisation and embryology authority – HFEA) to be ineffective.

Nevertheless, the journalist continues to be anxious about 'desperate' women who will 'humbly accept any risk, pay any price and endure almost any slight from the God like men who promise new life'.... Indeed, she is anxious about 'egg sharing', a widespread practice whereby poor women get subsidised treatment in return for their excess eggs which are implanted in women who no longer have eggs, described, somewhat disingenuously, by the journalist, as 'richer, older ones' (it's possible to become infertile quite young). 'Ovarian hyperstimulation' (the stimulation of the release of more eggs) was regarded also as a cause for concern but without explanation as to why, as was 'foetal reduction' (the removal of excess foetuses in cases when several eggs have been fertilised to reduce the possibility of miscarriage). The most wildly controversial thing she was worrying about was the 'discredited insistence on donor anonymity'. Why discredited? Can you imagine having a donor egg fertilised by your partner's sperm and then implanted in your uterus, being pregnant and giving birth, then to have some woman turning up in your life making claims on your child? If carrying a child to term and giving birth to it doesn't make it yours then nothing does! Conversely, can you imagine your pain if your child were to decide, on turning eighteen, to find out who his or her 'real' mother was. Yes, you bore the child but it's not your genetic material – you are not the 'real' mother. Can you imagine the absolute quagmire of misery that abandoning donor anonymity would produce? I can. Let's hope the new beefed up HFEA of the future makes the right decisions.

Monday 1st Sept 03.

Yesterday we went to Hillsborough Leisure Centre with the children, who absolutely adore it. Emile likes to potter round in the shallows, having inexplicably lost his former bravery. He squealed peevishly when I let him float by himself, supported by his little armbands – didn't like it at all. Eilish, in contrast, is now a "mermaid", having had two one-to-one swimming lessons with a very sweet young woman, called Nicci, at my health club. She insisted on swimming the entire length of the pool to the deep end. Although, I was right next to her, I was terrified she'd suddenly lose it, and sink like a stone, after all, it's just a question of will, this swimming business. But she was fine. She can swim.

It's day fourteen of my cycle and we had sex again, having decided, following yet another conversation on when to have coitus: to have sex every day from day 12 through to 16, if possible.

Tuesday 2nd Sept 03.
Today I was away from home so unable to procreate. For one reason or another, we don't seem to manage the run through my potentially fertile days. I suppose I could have taken some sperm with me in a little jar or something, but I'm assuming there is still some lurking about ready to do the business.

Wednesday 3rd Sept 03.
Today Emile did a lovely thing for the first time. I was sitting on the floor and I opened my arms to him. Instead of waddling up to me, he ran into my arms with complete abandon. Then he walked backwards across the room and ran into my arms again with the same level of absolute enthusiasm and unalloyed joy. Then he walked backwards and did the same thing again, and again, and again. It was beautiful.
Our au-pair, Maristella, who has a philosophical streak, noted in her thick Brazilian accent, "look you can't buy this for money; this is real happiness…" I certainly can't imagine not having children.
It's day 16 of my cycle today so it's possible I could be having a late ovulation. Nevertheless, we were both too knackered to have sex by the time we were snuggled up in bed. We just cuddled and talked, but I can't help wondering how many fertile cycles I have left… I am actually, feeling broody now. I think Robert had been broody continuously but it's just hitting me now – now I've had time to forget the birth pain.

Thursday – Sunday 4-7th Sept 03.
I've been busy with my work and preparations for selling my cottage in Derbyshire – collating documents for my solicitor, finding a storage company, getting quotes for removals, commissioning a structural survey of the property we're buying, corresponding about fixtures and fittings and a complication about the ground lease, seeing an independent mortgage advisor, getting a bridging loan from Robert's parents and so forth. It's all surprisingly time consuming.

I spent the morning in the park with the children, which was pleasant and uneventful, apart from a particularly spectacular tantrum by Emile. It was a lying on his back, thrashing his limbs and screaming tantrum, but neither he, nor I, are quite sure why he had it. Fortunately, I've reached a point where this no longer embarrasses or distressed me. He was laughing and cheerful again within three minutes.

Wednesday 10th Sept 03.

I managed to get around to watching the latest episode of *Sex and the City, 'Hop, Skip and a Week'*. In this episode being a mother in a pressurised job is explored. Miranda, the lawyer, is seen leaving for work. Magda, her nanny, holds the crying infant and the voice over tells us "along with her coffee, feeling guilty had become part of Miranda's daily routine". When at work Miranda is hauled into her manager's office; there are two senior managers there – always a bad sign. It's noted that she's been struggling to handle her caseload and that she has arrived late, rather frequently, for meetings. She gives a spirited response, saying that the lateness won't happen again but reminding them that she is doing a good job – indeed, the only place where she is doing a bad job, she asserts, is as a mother.

Later she is seen arriving home and asking Magda, her nanny, if the baby is still awake. So many times I've rushed home myself to find Eilish fast asleep. I've sat in traffic jams yearning to cuddle her. So I could relate to Miranda's disappointment on being told that he'd been asleep for sometime. Indeed, these are the moments which convince us that we pay a very high price for our careers. Being conscientious, Miranda shrugs off her disappointment and gets on with some work she's brought home with her; however, the next day she is seen telling her boss that she must reduce her hours to a 50-hour week.

Personally, I think I'm seen as a bit of a slacker by some of my colleagues as I put in less 'face-time' than some others. I spend on average only 25-30 hours a week in my office. I work between a 37 and a 47 hour week in total, but that doesn't include all the work related reading I do, which probably accounts for a further ten hours.

Thursday 11th Sept 03.

I wanted to explain to Robert how trying to become pregnant makes me feel emotionally vulnerable. "Well I understand you could die", he offered. I explained that it's changed my relationship to my body – that I'm constantly scrutinising myself – constantly interrogating my bodily experience for signs of fertility or conception. I explained that when I am trying to conceive I feel very emotionally open to him and that I am therefore exceptionally sensitive to his mood swings or him being slightly terse. I find I can't create emotional distance when I might be carrying his child.

I tried to talk about my fears: I feel very ill when pregnant (perhaps this one could be worse than the last), I lose my intellectual ability (with my first pregnancy I felt the very essence of who I am was being annihilated). In less optimistic moments, I worry that I could end up Caesarean Sectioned or haemorrhaging.

I also wonder if it's stopping me enjoying my children as much as I might if I knew for certain I wasn't going to have another. When I had Eilish, I thought she'd be an only child so I really gave myself up to her in a way I simply haven't with Emile. Not that there aren't moments of surrender. My surrender to him, that is. There are plenty and they feel precious; however, I now sit snatching moments with my P.C. rather than with my twenty-month-old baby with the assumption that there will be another baby for me to experience.

If all goes well, we have a new house. A few nights ago I realised there was no obvious place to have the baby in the new house. Here we've got a fairly large bathroom. I thought I'd just run a bath and hop in. There's room for the midwives and Robert to attend me.

My last birth lasted 1 hour and 25 minutes from first contraction to babe in arms, so I was thinking of something along the following lines. When the waters break Robert would make me a couple of cups of tea while I relax in bed. After drinking lots of liquids, I'd then try to empty my bowels. Once the contractions get close together I'd hop in the bath and Robert will phone the midwives. They'd arrive just in time to check the baby over on its arrival, but would keep a discreet distance while Robert delivered the baby. The last sentence is pure fantasy, of course.

Now, in the new house there's a miniscule bathroom and I know the community midwives won't agree to my labouring in it. They'll insist, quite reasonably, on having a bit of room to move. Given the mess involved, I don't want to give birth in a bedroom. There's a big laundry in the new house so I guess I'd have to make that space viable somehow. I was hoping to use a bath rather than have to construct a birth pool – the idea of using a bath was partly to avoid getting sucked into all the politics again. Many midwives are edgy about pool births, for no good reason (I'm an academic and I've looked up the recent papers in the British Medical Journal on the *theoretical possibility* of water embolism). In Edinburgh, where I had Eilish, it was fine to have the first and second stages of labour in the pool (the baby and then the placenta) but in Derbyshire, where I was registered for number two, they didn't want the second stage in the water. AIMS (the Association for Improvements in Midwifery Services) told me it was *my right* to do as I wanted. That was why both Robert and a friend, experienced in attending homebirths, had been lined up to give me support. They were supposed to tell the midwives calmly and politely how things were going to be... Anyway, I know that as soon as I mention the words 'birth pool', I'm going to get a reaction, so leaping into the bath instead seemed a more relaxing option.

Friday 12th September 03.
Today was Robert's thirty-third birthday. My 'toy-boy' is ageing. I took him out to *Candytown*, which boasts the best Chinese food in Sheffield (though it's just been refurbished in such a ugly manner I'm not sure I'll be able to bring myself to eat there again). At the table next to us was a family with four children – not bickering. Robert spent the evening bloodily glancing at their toddler (slightly younger than ours). I wish I could have told him I was pregnant for his birthday.

Saturday 13th September 03.
There was an article in *The Guardian* Weekend magazine today, a re-hash of Hewlitt's *Baby Hunger* thesis, entitled *The Generation that Took a Gamble*. What it should have been called is *Get On With It*. It featured discussion about women who left it 'perilously, and unnecessarily late' to try and conceive children. The author, Joanna Briscoe, (who had her first baby at the age of 37) is worried about a whole load of thirty-something women out there who are 'bewilderingly casual in their approach to possible parenthood.' Her message is mate before it's too late. Although

the author claims not to be one of those sniggering 'at all [the] withered old career bitches for being so selfish', the tone of her piece is nevertheless quite reactionary, suggesting that women have to choose between home and work.

I'm not sure many women of my generation really thought they could fit having children 'seamlessly' into our lives, as she suggests – that's precisely why we put it off, and put it off, and off. Personally, I married someone who didn't want children and only after about a decade of marriage did I realise he really meant it. Lots of my friends had married men who didn't want children either but who had all 'cracked'. Some of them said they'd never own a house: 'property is theft', after all, or a car: one should use public transport. But by this point they all had mortgages, kids and cars.

According to the article, the majority of late in life mothers claim that the reason they did not have children earlier is because they had not met the right person to have them with (this is just gracious, isn't it?). Briscoe suggests that this 'lack of a partner' problem is due to women being too fussy: 'We feel we fall short if we don't manage to find a sensitive specimen of a Heathcliffian lover who will later prove to be a model of paternal perfection…' I think this is absolute bollocks but the message is clear. You see, all we women have to do is lower our expectations and pick a nice bloke who'll do his share of the childcare. It's our desires which are at fault. Unfortunately, this doesn't really take into account that we might want different things from men (or one man) at different points in our lives. In our early twenties perhaps it's a passionate lover we want, whether or not he likes children might seem irrelevant from that vantage point. Hewlett's suggestion that women be 'tactical' in their thirties about finding a partner and having children wasn't *instead* of having a career or a satisfying relationship. Her research on professional women indicated that high achieving women are happier if they stay in work after having children, though this may be on a reduced hours contract. Her research also indicates that high achieving women want to be with other high achievers – people they can relate to, rather than lower paid, possibly more domesticated, men.

The role of men wasn't explored at all in the piece. Until it becomes socially acceptable for men to take serious quantities of parental leave, parenting career breaks, to demand reduced hours contacts or flexi-time because they are parents, it's going to remain tough on women. The big breakthrough for women will come when parenting becomes genuinely more shared.

The good thing about the piece, though it made us older 'dinosaurs' seem rather grotesque, is that it's positive about motherhood. The author's take on the subject is: 'Nothing can prepare you for the exhausting drudgery; nothing can prepare you for the transcendent joy.' One of the interviewees, Clover Hughes, said: "Because motherhood is such a wonderful experience, surely that's something you would want to do earlier on in your life? I think people don't realise how nice it is. It's been a huge joy." That seems the best point on which to end.

Sunday 14th September 03.

The Observer Magazine had a piece by Barbara Ellen about the birth of her tiny premature baby (3lb 3oz) born by emergency Caesarean Section at London's Chelsea and Westminster Hospital. It had Asymmetrical Inter-Uterine Growth Retardation (AIUGR) preferable to other varieties of the disorder, because the brain in prioritised by the failing placenta. That's a nice way of saying that it's probably not brain damaged though all its other organs will be very underdeveloped. The baby is now fine, and very beautiful it has to be said.

The article reminded me a lot of my friend Becky's recent experience of having a very premature baby by emergency Caesarean. She too had to wait for hours (though in a wheelchair with her catheter bunged up) for someone to come so she could see her baby. She too had to beg for a busy nurse to wheel her over to her daughter's incubator. I wondered if it was the same hospital. Ellen said of her experience: 'No one was expecting a stay at the Waldorf, but you couldn't help but notice the blood-stained bed linen, dirty lavatories, unanswered bells and small minority of surly neglectful nurses.' When her husband returned a few hours later he found her: 'drenched in sweat, unable to stop shaking and crying.'

Monday 15th September 03.

In *Sex and the City*, an episode entitled *'The Post-it Always Sticks Twice'*, Miranda despondently bemoans the fact that clubs are for "hot" childless people. I happen to know that's a myth because Robert takes me to some of these young persons' clubs and bars (as I think of them) and they are full of glamorous or slutty, scantily dressed young women (half my age) and a wide variety of men. Many of the women are notable for how little they are wearing. The men vary from testosterone-spewing packs of working class males wearing the uniform pastel coloured shirts (even in the dead of winter) to the gigolo types (lone males or in pairs) who will grope a women's bum almost immediately he starts talking to her, to test whether or not he'll get his 'leg-over' later. Amazingly, I've seen a woman having her bum groped by one of these specimens only to see the same woman having her bum groped by a different man about an hour later! There are also small groups of geeks who look like they will never have the courage to talk to a woman. And there are gays, out and relaxed and mingling. Very rarely do I see a man I'd be interested in, though occasionally there's a hot young Asian who'll catch my eye. I like pretty boys. Anyway, the point I was going to make was that in the ladies' loo these women are always having loud drunken conversations as they share a cubicle or chat in the queue and I have overheard loads of conversations about children, childcare, their children's access arrangements with ex-husbands and partners and so on. These very young slutty girls, getting their arses groped, are mums. Well, some of them certainly are.

So back to *Sex and the City,* Miranda is feeling negative until she discovers she is thin enough to squeeze into her pre-pregnancy jeans. She's stopped having time to eat as a busy single mum we are told (ignore all the previous episodes featuring her eating chocolate cake in front of the TV). They go to a club called *'Bed' (*which does have beds rather than chairs to sit on). Miranda is chatted up almost immediately and realises she is sexually attractive (and hasn't got 'single-mum' tattooed on her forehead) – it's all a question of attitude.

Tuesday 16th September 03.

I just came across a piece about babies smiling in the womb, caught by the latest scanning equipment. I thought the extraordinary thing about the article was obstetrician's observation about smiling, which I assumed to be one of a number of bodily reflexes played out in-utero, linked to cognitive development. Stuart Campbell said, 'It is remarkable that a newborn baby does not smile for about six weeks after birth. But before birth, most babies smile frequently. This may indicate the baby's trouble-free existence in the womb and the relatively traumatic first few weeks after birth when the baby is reacting to a strange environment.' Interesting.

Sunday 21th September 03.
In *Sex and the City ('The Catch')* Miranda, who has had a baby with Steve but is not living with him, receives a gift from Steve's girlfriend: aromatherapy oils for serenity and calm. Presumably, she thinks that's what Miranda needs, based on Steve's account of her. Can they become friends? The answer seems to be no. When Steve, girlfriend in tow, turn up to collect baby Brady, Miranda hides under the cot to avoid meeting her. She's not in a position to "let go" of her feelings about Steve because they have a baby – though the suggestion of the slightly ambiguous text is that she should be able to do this.

Wednesday 24th September 03.
Eilish smashed me in the face with a toy today and I smacked her and sent her to her room where she cried in a histrionic fashion for over half-an-hour. I felt really terrible, not for shouting or sending her to her room but for the slap. I went out for the evening. Maristella, who put her to bed, told me she was really sad and kept telling her "I love my mummy…"

Thursday 25th September 03.
It's vinegar douche time (an extra weak solution, just in case that is why I haven't conceived yet). I've just seen two jobs I'd like to apply for but when I imagine I could be impregnated at any moment it seems positively irresponsible to apply. Both are research fellowships so the intellectual atrophy, which seems to afflict me during pregnancy, would be particularly unwelcome and disruptive. At least in my current job, I managed to bumble my way through my familiar teaching, albeit in an uninspirational fashion, more or less adequately. Actually, I was exhausted the whole time and now think it's quite inhumane to make pregnant women work at all. I wrote quite a bad essay later in the pregnancy, which unfortunately is in the public domain. No doubt someone will use it against me at some point (that's what academics are like).

Robert was aloof and busy earlier which hasn't really put me in the mood to have sex with him. Perhaps I'll be able to regain my loving feelings by bedtime.

Friday 26th September 03.

Well the sex last night was great. I like sex! I abhor the thought of our relationship becoming just domestic. Today Maristella has to go off to try to sort out matters regarding her visa. She will not return until Sunday. Emile is such an incredibly undemanding baby. I got to watch lots of programmes on TV that I'd heard about but not seen before, including *Judge Judy*, a wonderful North American import showing a real judge at work with petty felons. He pottered about quite contentedly, occasionally requesting that I put a shape in the correct position. By far his favourite toys are these wooden shapes that slot into a board. He's got lots of these because he likes them so much, and will literally spend two hours at a time putting the bits in the correct places and then rearranging them. Having noticed that these were his favourite toys, I bought him some interactive ones with sheep that bleat, or cows that moo and so forth, when assigned to their correct position, but strangely he doesn't like these better than the others. The obsession is clearly about shapes and their placement rather than the meanings of the objects. It's a pleasure just to watch him play.
The other thing he likes to do is simply to move piles of things from one place to another. In the garden after lunch it was spadefulls of sand – but it could have been anything. He had a little bounce on his trampoline, sat on the trike (which he hasn't worked out how to propel yet), and in his toy car, even did some pretend cooking at Eilish's toy kitchen. Then at 1.30 he let me put him in his cot for his afternoon nap without complaint, such a happy little baby. Eilish always cried when I put her down to sleep – they could not have been more different temperamentally. I blame my lack of experience with babies, not her genes, for the differences between them. Emile is relaxed because I am relaxed.

Sunday 28th September 03.

I've had a miserable weekend (with some good bits relating to the children). I don't know if I'm more volatile and sensitive because I'm getting 'cold feet' before the big commitment (we are due to buy a house together in a fortnight) but I have found Robert bullish, aggressive, abrasive, argumentative and hard to be around. He says he's tense and will be different in the new house because he'll be relaxed then. I say, "jam tomorrow". I want him to demonstrate he can be a loving sensitive partner now.

In *Sex and the City ('A Woman's Right to Shoes')* Carrie Bradshaw, who has an obsession with over-priced footwear, loses her shoes at a friend's party. Well, 'loses' is unfair. They were either mistakenly taken by another partygoer or stolen by someone who recognised them as incredibly expensive footwear.

When she tells her friend she shrugs, and suggests they'll turn up. Carrie is distraught and obsesses about her designer footwear. She's upset that here friend was so blasé. After all this is EXPENSIVE DESIGNER FOOTWEAR we are talking about. When she tells the girls about the incident she even tots up all the money she'd spent on her friend over the years: wedding gifts, kids birthdays etc. – it adds up to more than the replacement value of her shoes. (The host should have whipped out her chequebook obviously). Of her 'friend' she says, "she's had two Caesareans and a lobotomy" (ouch). This gives Samantha her cue for an anti-children diatribe… "I'm so sick of these people with their children… they're everywhere, sitting next to me in first class, eating at the next table…." Samantha would like to see them segregated by legislation, presumably.

Later in the programme, Samantha, having been told by a waiter she can't use her mobile phone in a restaurant, asks the waiter if he can do anything about "that noise", indicating a child at a nearby table. No, is the answer. When she inadvisably decides to take matters into her own hands, the child throws spaghetti at her. Good for you kid was my response.

Anyway, Carrie decides to confront her friend about the missing shoes. She calls round at the friend's home and asks if they have been returned. She's polite and sheepish but the penny-drops and the girlfriend realises she is supposed to whip out her checkbook. The host is apologetic – of course she should have offered to replace them. How much should she make the cheque payable for? When Carrie says $485.00 dollars her friend thinks she's joking.

She's not joking of course (in an earlier episode she tots up that she has spent $40,000 on her wardrobe of shoes). She has been obsessing about these shoes. Her friend says feels uncomfortable subsidising her "extravagant" life-style. She is "crazy" to pay so much for shoes (so far, I'm with the friend) but then she gets preachy: Yes, she too may have been extravagant in the past, "before I had a real life" she asserts, before she had meaningful "responsibilities". Carrie is exposed as an inane bimbo and the friend as a hypocrite – They are "just shoes", points out her friend. Later her friend is described as a "fucking bitch" for having made Carrie feel shameful about her, to my mind, absurd infatuation with the shoes. Carrie worries that we are not "celebrating each other's life choices", which sounds like a phrase from pop-psychology. I'm not sure people in developing countries watching their children die, needlessly, of diarrhoea because of polluted water supplies, would celebrate Carrie's particular life-choice.

When she phones her 'friend' some days later she realises, whilst she has been dwelling on the incident, her friend has been busy with her children and hasn't given the matter a second thought. The matter is resolved in the end when Carrie leaves a voice-message telling her friend where she can buy her a gift (surprise, surprise) of very expensive shoes. Somewhat implausibly, the busy friend does trot along and pay for these. So the episode has a happy ending and a warm message about tolerance of each other's "life-choices". I'm not sure that this really reflects what is happening in America where increasingly intolerant 'child-free' workers are organising against parents who they see as getting more company perks. Conversely, I think the busy mum might have done better to have dumped Carrie from her social circle rather than pay almost 500 bucks on shoes.

Thursday 2nd October 03.

When I was packing up my old house I came across some interviews I'd done in 1996 with a Ph.D. student who was conducting a study on attitudes to home births. I haven't looked at all the material yet but it was interesting to re-visit my old self. At 26 weeks pregnant, I sound very tired. I talk about my desire to have a home-birth. At one point I say that I think I'll be able to use my experience of meditating to help control the pain, and my anxiety about the pain. How calm and optimistic I sound!

In the event, it was a long and excruciating labour and whilst I did hold-up for quite a long time, I eventually succumbed to the incredible intensity of the pain and rising feelings of panic. My second labour was even more intense and the pain and the terror engulfed me almost immediately, but it was mercifully brief and without the terrible side effects of the perineum tearing, as it did with the first.

Friday 3th October 03.
I'm not losing enthusiasm for keeping this diary except that every spare moment I get, and I guess I should have inverted commas around the word 'spare', I'm spending sorting out all the house business. I'm selling next week, buying the week after (except that the upward 'chain' is threatening to 'break' – in other words, someone is threatening to pull out). I'm changing agent for my Scottish house (also for sale). It is all immeasurably time consuming and stressful. The owners of Collegiate Crescent (the house we hope to buy) have been haggling over the price of fixtures and fittings, which has necessitated my making a further visit to the property. Robert has just sold the house I'm sitting in, so, if there are unforeseen delays with the purchase, I guess we could end up in rented accommodation.
The idea is that we sell our houses and buy one big family house. The house in question, described (incorrectly) as a 'dress stone double-fronted Georgian residence', is early Victorian; but it's massive and gives us a playroom, guest room, two lounges as well as bedrooms for the au-pair, ourselves, and two children. The feature that Eilish likes the best was the fort in the garden built by the current architect owner. That caused its own problems, as it does not meet normal building regulations… I had to be willing to accept a disclaimer…

Saturday 4th October 03.
This week's *Guardian* Weekend magazine had a huge piece on a woman who has written a novel exploring a mother's feelings of abhorrence towards her child. The author, Lionel Shriver, is childless, though, to give Shriver credit, the quotes of her writing indicate a forceful use of language. Nevertheless, I do wonder why I should be interested in a childless woman's dark fantasies about motherhood. The mother is a

'haggard cow' and her breast milk 'nauseating'. The child grows up and commits violent atrocities that are perhaps the result of the mother's attitude towards her offspring (such mother blaming is by no means original or new).

In her interview with Rachael Cusk the author admits to an absolute "horror" of being pregnant. What was very telling was her dismissal of mothers who told her that they felt motherhood 'rejuvenated your life at its core' – which I think it does, except that it tires you out simultaneously. She says in interview that she's heard that kind of claim so often that it begins to "ring a little hollow". I thought that quite a bizarre statement (and unfortunately Cusk doesn't challenge her). Surely, women keep saying it because that's their experience – because it's true.

The author says that the son (Kevin) reinforces the mother's dislike of herself and takes away the things she likes about herself. The author suggests that all parents can recognise this; however, I can't relate to this. Yes, my need to be in control is highlighted by some of my interactions with my children. But I can successfully control this impulse to be in control. This makes me feel good about myself, incidentally. Likewise, my irritation at their wanting to sniff a flower when I am marching us off to catch a bus is confronted and I relax. I miss the bus. I see the flower. I appreciate the moment. I feel that my children bring out **the best in me** and **highlight what is really important** – the moment, the here and now. There is a huge gulf that exists between women with children and women without children. Shriver at 47 has probably missed her chance to become a mother. Her neurotic fantasies might help console childless women, or women who feel phobic about motherhood, that they've made the right decision, but it's important to recognise that this is fiction we are talking about.

Sunday 5th October 03.

We slept over at my Derbyshire cottage, which is due to be sold next week. Yesterday Robert and I revisited all the places we used to go when we started dating. Today Eilish went to say goodbye to the park in which she spent so much of her time, when younger.

Tuesday 7th October 03.

I stayed over in Derbyshire to pack-up the house and then did my normal sleep-over on Monday so I didn't get to see the children until tonight. Emile was fine, as usual. But Eilish was a bit weepy and I wondered if it was to do with her emotions about saying goodbye to our old life together in Derbyshire.

Sunday 12th October 03.

I went to see a film about the Israeli occupation of the West Bank, called *Jeremy Hardy Versus the Israeli Army*. Hardy is a quirky British stand-up comedian. He ends up in Bethlehem in April 2002, just before the siege of the nativity. What really amazed me was an Israeli tank firing on the Palestinian maternity hospital and machine-gunning the statue of the Virgin Mary, which stands its courtyard. Clearly, no one is safe in Bethlehem.

Saturday 18th October 03.

I just read such an irritating piece in the *Guardian* that I have to write a riposte. Hopefully, it will be published next weekend. As sent:

Zoe Doesn't Get It.

It is a platitude to insist that nothing can prepare us for the intensity and power of motherhood, but it is also true. I was bemused by Zoe Williams's rant, *'The Parent Trap'*, in *The Guardian* Weekend (18.10.03.). Where to start in the morass of misconceptions? No, Zoe having children is NOT like having siblings. When you idealise children you 'undermine the value of complexity and of challenge', she asserts. Perhaps, but then again, maybe you appreciate simplicity. Perhaps you appreciate the moment, a moment you might have missed had you not been in a child's presence. You can be complex and challenged another time and in a different context. (Caesareans and lobotomies aren't automatically performed together, Zoe – such old-fashioned sexism from a *Guardian* writer makes me disappointed).

Whilst women have different responses to motherhood, dependent on their circumstances and personality, no doubt there are a few who are revoltingly smug; however, it is absurd and unhelpful to suggest that mothers 'attack' non-mothers in general. Zoe Williams's hostile generalisations invite such attack though, especially in the context of a recent spate of anti-motherhood articles written by childless women. Why is it okay for these childless women to trot-out what used to be called misogyny? Williams's cant invites reductive responses.

Her generalisations about childless women being 'infantilised' are ridiculous. It's possible that the reluctance of doctors to sterilise relatively young women is based purely on medical grounds, it being an *irreversible procedure* in many cases, and nothing to do with the idea that women are not seen as mature until they have had children. Personally, I became more infantile after having children in that I became more in touch with the irrational bits of myself I could see being expressed in my children. I became less restrained generally – more playful in fact…

What Zoe Williams illustrates is she doesn't understand that motherhood alters everything – all our relationships. To give a simple example, before having children I used to sit anonymous and silent on the bus. I was the kind of person you'd see reading a book. After having my baby, I was drawn into conversation with a multitude of women I had **never even noticed before**. All the conversations centred on my baby. This happened all the time and ***completely transformed*** my experience of using public transport. That's a trivial example, all key relationships in my life changed (not always in ways that I liked). Long buried feelings about my relationship with my parents surfaced. My emotional perception of myself changed. My feelings about my employment changed and my employer's attitude to me shifted too. There was loss too (and Rachael Cusk is good on this point) in having to amend and truncate my life to fit around child-care schedules. Goodbye spontaneity (at least after the second). And not being able to attend that conference in Madrid or snap up that cheap flight to Barcelona never gets less frustrating… But the pay-off is profound, Zoe, and perhaps unimaginable to you 'child-free'…

I showed the letter to Robert. He said that they'd never print it because it's much too long.

Sunday 19th October 03.

Feeling tempted to send this to *The Observer*, in which the offending piece appeared.

Rose, We Mothers Don't Think Childless Women are Selfish Bitches

(though a few may be).

The media is becoming obsessed with motherhood (ironically, in a week in which fathers are due to take to the street to demand more rights over their offspring). It's predicted (by whom it is not said) that by 2010 about 22% of British women will be childless. There is a decline in the birth rate in Britain, and lots of other places besides, and only child-friendly and family-friendly policies will be able to halt this trend. I look forward to being able to tax-deduct my childcare costs, as it is possible to do in many other countries. If Tony Blair *really* wanted women to work he'd have allowed us to do this ages ago. In *Happily Unblessed*, a number of childless women make rather bland remarks about not having children. These range from it being a 'non-issue' to rather silly remarks about babies being an 'accessory'. Well, then it's an accessory that demands almost constant attention. Anyone with experience of looking after babies must find this notion of the baby as a passive object ridiculous (they only stay still in the photographs, love). Babies revolt the author but most of the interviewees quite liked children. 'Wilful non-parenting,' asserts Rose Shepherd, is '*just not on.*' While I'm very sorry to hear that Rose once had a bad experience at a dinner party, at which a mother insulted her as being selfish for not having children, I have to say that her assumption that mothers in general feel antagonistic to non-mothers is just paranoia. Not liking babies is a cliché rather than 'heresy', I'd suggest. Turn on *Sex and the City* and Samantha will tell you how much she dislikes children in almost every episode.

Rose suggests that 'There are other, maybe better things to bequeath to posterity than your progeny – other, and maybe better ways of realising your purpose, and of assuring your immortality'. Having children wasn't about achieving 'immortality' for me. It was about wanting to have a relationship with a child and then children. And, Rose, please remember it's not actually an and/or choice. Mothers can make a contribution to posterity **and** raise children. This *leit-motif* in recent articles that motherhood renders women dumb or unambitious is offensive.

Monday 20th October 03.

This is the night I sleep in another city and I was feeling very sexually frustrated. It's only day 12 of my cycle. I've also been feeling broody, as the daughter of my host is pregnant so our mealtime conversation kept returning to this topic. She's a Muslim, so I must ask her about birthing practices in her community.

Tuesday 21st October 03.
When I got back Robert and I made love and I had a titanic orgasm. I must be ovulating quite early in my cycle.

Wednesday 22nd October 03.
Robert jumped on me again this morning before he went to work. I think it's because we'd been cuddling and he'd happened to get an erection rather than him being utterly determined to impregnate me this month.

Thursday 23rd October 03.
I managed to get around to watching *Sex and the City*, an episode called *'The Domino Effects'* in which Charlotte has acupuncture to increase her chances of conception. Then she miscarries and is very despondent. Meanwhile, Miranda, who is dating a 'hot' hunky and charismatic doctor realises that she can't say the words, *I love you.* He has declared his love to Miranda, somewhat implausibly, on a cookie (perhaps Americans do do this kind of thing…). He'd arrived with pizza and inscribed cookie at Miranda's apartment; however, being a doctor, his pager goes off, as they do, and Miranda is confronted with the *I love you* cookie alone. Surely, she can pluck up the courage to tell him she loves him too? After all, he is "perfect". He's "hot" and sweet with her son, Brady. Meanwhile, the distinctly unmaternal Samantha has found a grey hair in her pubic hair. She is dismayed, as "no man wants to fuck grandma's pussy".
Miranda confides to her friends that she's incapable of opening herself emotionally to a man. She feels she is going to ruin her life. She'll never have intimacy. She can't say the words…
During Brady's first birthday party she finds herself alone with Steve (Brady's father), whilst they put candles in the cake. Suddenly, in an unexpected twist of the plot, she declares her love for him and he responds positively. It looks as though they are going to ditch their respective partners (both of whom will be devastated) and get back together again.

Steve tells her you are "the one". The biological parents will be reunited.

Friday 24th October 03.
We 'completed' on the house yesterday and Robert will oversee the move while I'm at work on Monday (he has ten days holiday whereas I have none). Consequently, I have only one more day of normal routine in this house for on Sunday I must pack.
I took Eilish to see the new house in the evening and she was delighted with the little wooden fort in the garden. She wasn't particularly interested in anything else except the pull-out 'pantry unit' in the kitchen. She was slightly dismayed to learn that we weren't going to get all the nice furniture we'd seen when viewing.
Robert and I had intercourse in the morning (not inspired love making – what Robert calls a "quick fuck") and, in the evening, although he was enthusiastic to pleasure me, he was unable to get an erection, despite my giving him encouragement! I doubt at day 16 whether I'm still fertile so I was happy to relax and enjoy non-penetrative sex. Nevertheless, I do wonder about his lack of stamina!

Saturday 25th October 03.
I had a lovely time in the morning with the children. I actually had both children on my lap looking at a storybook together (for the first time). I much prefer to try to create a tranquil atmosphere. Emile is capable of pottering about in a gentle manner. Eilish can be very peaceful.
Maristela, on the other hand, is tremendously energetic, she has the TV turned up loud or plays pop music, she moves around a lot from room to room slamming doors, she is happy to have them practising gymnastics on the sofas! She has a restless disposition. The shrieking and crashing is abominable. Both she and Robert even speak loudly. The children get overexcited and Emile throws his bricks, hits or bites Eilish. Tears ensue. This isn't at all what I envisaged.
I like Maristela. She is good fun, and we are even going dancing together at the Juju Club next Wednesday, but I hope her replacement will have a sensitive disposition and a serene manner… Having someone like Maristela around all the time is wearing.
In the afternoon I took Eilish to see the new house again. Since it's got a

“castle” in the garden, I don’t think she’ll be nostalgic about leaving this house.

Sunday 26th October 03.
I’m feeling quite traumatised at the prospect of having to pack up my computer. Furthermore, I’ve got a bad cold. To my left is a large stack of boxes which I must fill.

Tuesday 4th November 03.
I’m writing from my new desk in my new room in the new house. I’m feeling slightly disorientated. Today was a strange day partly because of all the explosions going off all the time, which make me jumpy. Why can’t everyone bloody well ignite their fireworks on Guy Fawkes’ Day. Also, I had to drive home in the dark which is a peculiar form of sensory deprivation, as the drive takes 90 minutes. The huge Victorian windows in our new house flood with light at 6.00am, or so, which wakes me up at a time I’d like to be sleeping.
Tonight Robert was sulky because he couldn’t work out how to make the oven work (the electricity had been switched off earlier) so we couldn’t have Nan bread with the Dahl (the slightest little thing seems to spoil his mood). At least the faulty boiler has been mended so it’s lovely and warm. Even my period didn’t come at its usual time. I started bleeding yesterday. I wonder if this is the beginning of menopause. Better have sex from day ten as presumably when I have these much shorter cycles I’m ovulating earlier.

Wednesday 5th October 03.
I am finally alone. Robert is at work, Eilish at school, Emile at his childminder and Maristella has gone out. The quiet is unfamiliar. I’ve been thinking about a piece on the radio news I heard last night, during my long drive along the dark duel carriageway, about a man called David Chick who has suspended himself from a crane in central London. He is protesting about lack of rights for fathers. Firstly, I will use inverted commas around the word ‘fathers’, because the word is used indiscriminately to mean any man who had impregnated a woman, even through rape. Apparently, *Fathers for Justice*, a campaigning organisation

for 'fathers', who organised the stunt, are trying to persuade him to come down but he's refusing. Presumably, since he's been selected for this stunt, he's reasonably 'clean'. But I do wonder what he has done which makes a woman who once had sex with him not want him to have any access to the progeny of that union? Was he violent towards the child or the mother? Was he otherwise abusive? Did he smash up the furniture in temper tantrums? Did he steal her things to fund his drug habit? Was he a liar who cheated on her who she thinks will be a bad influence on the child? How bad was he? Now I'm desperate to find out their story.

Although, when Robert has been cruel or insensitive to me, I have threatened to leave (and when we were weekending together I flounced off a couple of times) I cannot really imagine taking the children away from him. I feel tied to him through the children now. I just wonder how appalling these men are who have been rejected so resolutely.

Whilst I can perfectly understand a woman who conceives during casual sex not wanting a stranger interfering in her life, on the other hand, to leave the father of ones' child, in a long-term relationship, is not something that any mother would do lightly.

Thursday 6th November 03.

The news had no mention of men on cranes – very frustrating!

Wednesday 12th November 03.

Day 10 of my fertility cycle. Robert did his 'suck-fuck' thing: penetrative sex followed by cunnilingus followed by entry followed by cunnilingus, and so on. It's 100% successful in giving me orgasms – just a tip for male readers…

Thursday 13th November 03.

Although I was tired after my long day at the University I douched and then we had sex.

I guess we both really do want another child. I got very aroused in the end.

Friday 14th November 03.

Today is day 12 of my cycle, which because it's become shorter, is now my fertile day I think.

I spent the day working on a book I doubt I'll finish if I get pregnant again. I'm 42 years old so if I get pregnant my emphasis will be: rest, rest, and rest... I don't want to end up exhausted or ill.
There is the practical aspect of what to say to my publisher. I'm in the process of negotiating a contact. In my first correspondence with the series editor I put 18 months for the proposed delivery date, then I changed it to 2 years. Now I'm wondering if I should try to insert some sort of clause: 2 years but if I get pregnant, three. In my experience, publishers can get very stroppy if deadlines are not met but I know if I get pregnant I won't be able to finish it in time if they press for the deadline because of production schedules. In fact, I'm wildly behind my own schedule.

Saturday 15th November 03.
We missed having sex last night. Today is day 13 of my cycle so I might be ovulating. I feel sorry to have missed a day.

Sunday 16th November 03.
Last night both of us were exhausted but managed to 'make out'. I guess we do want this baby.
In the morning, I took Nolwenn, our new utterly delightful au-pair, and the children to the botanical gardens where Emile, in particular, was entranced by a couple of almost tame squirrels which approached us sniffing about his feet, his hands, but declining to eat the parsnip crisps he offered, then they actually followed us, repeatedly running up to Emile and Eilish. It was a beautiful sunny morning and the children really enjoyed looking at the squirrels and plants. We were just leaving the hot houses when Emile spied a tangerine, belonging to the packed lunch of one of the gardeners who were watering at the time. He pointed at it and said "mine". When I wouldn't give it to him he threw himself on the ground and thrashed and sobbed with such ferocity that I momentarily thought of stealing the bloody tangerine! Fancy leaving tempting tangerines lying about where toddlers can see them, how thoughtless! When he throws himself down in such abandoned despair I worry he will injure his face... Despite the tantrum, soon over, it was lovely to be in the sunshine.
In the evening we had sex again so that's days ten to fourteen (except twelve which we missed) 'done', so to speak, and tomorrow I'm sleeping

away so I'll be out of my possible ovulation period by my return on Tuesday.

Tuesday 18th November 03.
One of my students is heavily pregnant and in a small group tutorial today I found myself sitting with my tummy sticking out. I don't mean out of my garments, just puffed out a bit – you know the way pregnant women sit! (It's called, in psychological jargon, 'empathetic mirroring'). Fortunately, I managed to pull myself in before anyone noticed…

Wednesday 19th November 03.
Robert made a couple of telling remarks today. When I was depreciating myself for not looking after Eilish's hair well enough, having just lovingly combed and plaited it, I said: "my mother used to do this every morning for school", to which Robert responded, "your mother wasn't a Reader in Cultural Studies", invoking my professional status in support of my maternal failings; however, just a few hours earlier when I'd joked about my career progressively going down the drain as a result of my never getting any uninterrupted research time I'd been startled by his reply (unusually, my university doesn't support sabbaticals, except externally funded ones). I'd had a heating engineer in and a handyman in during my research time and the new au pair interrupted me umpteen times (the latter being fine, I expect to be on-hand for a new person). All the same, I'd ended up having another unproductive day and when I made my little quip Robert responded with, "what do you expect? You've got a family now. *You don't need a career…*!" Whilst I love my family, I'm not sure that it can obliterate my desire for some sort of career. I feel both simultaneously bolstered and deflated by Robert's remarks. Being a fundamentally provocative person, I countered with a remark that designed to tease, "you should have become an M.D. and then you could afford to keep me", though I'm not sure I would actually allow myself to be kept. Robert comes from a long line of highly successful medical doctors and his father, a consultant surgeon, was absolutely appalled when he declined to enter the family profession, especially in favour of a career in sports journalism! It was the cause of much friction between them for many years.

Thursday 20th November 03.

I'm finding it hard to write this diary when I'm feeling at all negative about my relationship with Robert. I guess it's because this image of us as a happy couple in our huge new luxurious family home with our lovely children feels like a public image, a construct, rather than a reality when the relationship starts to feel as though it's about to fragment.

Friday 21st November 03.

I am toiling with my research project and since I associate intellectual inertia with pregnancy I wonder if I am pregnant. This is the not knowing time of the month. I don't dwell on it but thoughts invade my consciousness. Today, I suddenly found myself wondering how my boss would react to hearing that I'm pregnant for the fourth time.

Saturday 22nd November 03.

Day 20 of my cycle. The final six to eight days seem to pass slowly as I await my fate. Emile, nearly 23 months, has started being incredibly affectionate. I think he's mimicking his sister a lot so now when I'm with him he wants to shower me with little kisses. Apart from the intermittent tantrum, throwing himself on his face and screaming, he has been utterly delightful. He's taken a couple of afternoon slots at the local nursery and was described as very sociable.

Sunday 23rd November 03.

I played my first game of Scrabble with Eilish today. I thought it might help her spelling. She played with Nolwenn's assistance with extra letters. And just as we begin to look like a well-organised and happy family in our new house, disaster strikes. The telephone rings and our new au pair is in tears. Nolwenn's mother's test results reveal that her cancer treatment is failing - a family friend phoning asked Nolwenn to come home immediately. My week is about to be dominated my another sort of scrabble – this one to patch together some sort of temporary childcare provision for Emile from the nursery (which only has the slots we've already got), other nurseries, local child minders, (if any have places), and baby sitters, plus chasing up the other young women who expressed interest in the au-pair post. In other words, it will be another week totally dominated by domestic affairs.

Monday 24th November 03.
I forgot to mention my little bedtime chat with Robert last night. It was one of those slightly bizarre chats which leave one with the unshakable opinion that ones partner is a lunatic. When I asked Robert why he'd seemed tense during both meal times me gave his usual, (and in itself totally unjustified, response for reasons I'll explain): "Because of Eilish". Eilish, let me tell you, is immensely well behaved at meal times, unlike Emile, who climbs out of his high chair if he can, balances precariously on any part of a chair or person's body, attempts to climb on to the table, takes food from other peoples plates, throws food or his drink cup, and runs round the table at high speed. He also recently stabbed himself in the face with a fork. Eilish, on the other hand, is polite, sits still and generally eats everything given to her. I pressed him further. At lunch he'd given her a smaller salad portion than usual (because she doesn't like it and because there wasn't much to go round); however, I'd eaten a piece from her plate (I don't usually eat from her plate, I was in a playful mood). Now, salad is the one food Eilish says she doesn't like and Robert insists she should learn to eat everything always gives her some – just because he's bloody-minded, I guess. His explanation for his tension: "I only gave her three lettuce leaves and you ate one". Okay? Did you get that? He was tense because I ate a lettuce leaf.
Okay, why was he tense at dinner? Was it because I'd eaten a Brussel-spout from her plate? No, it wasn't that, it was because she loves most of the food being served and "I was afraid she'd start asking about the potatoes", he said. "Afraid she'd start asking about the potatoes?", I was baffled. Eilish has sometimes asked why Robert he has six potatoes when she only has five, and such like audacious, but entirely unselfconscious questions, typical of those asked by six year olds. Such questions make him tense. On this occasion she asked no questions at all, but ***the mere thought that she might ask a question*** was enough to set him on edge for the entire meal. He is a lunatic isn't he? Please, someone, tell me I'm right! And of course I can get a bit tense too because he's being tense for reasons I can't discern and I'm wondering what's going on. I guess we should all go to family therapy. We need help don't we?

Tuesday 25th November 03.
Today I discovered that my application for a three-year research grant was unsuccessful. Putting together such applications represents a huge amount of hard work. The result means I won't be doing research for the next three years as I'd hoped. I felt quite tearful when I read the rejection letter. Later, in bed Robert suggested that I apply to work part-time and I agreed. He said that I should seek "satisfaction through my family" rather than through work. Again, I feel totally ambivalent about this, though perhaps some time out of full-time employment while the children are small won't do me any harm. On the other hand, quite a lot of research monies are only available to full-time academics (structurally academia is still geared up in favour of male careers with only a small percentage of women making it to the higher ranks of Reader or Professor: women accounting for about 15% of posts at this level), so I know I'll be cutting myself out of a lot of opportunities.

Wednesday 26th November 03.
On Monday I'd logged on to an au-pair web site I use. I e-mailed two likely candidates and luckily one of them, Sabrina, was on line at the time so we were able to have a detailed correspondence. She can join us next week. Nolwenn has chatted to her in French and thinks she is very nice, so it looks as though we've been lucky. That reminds me to check that Robert has phoned her referees…

Friday 28th November 03.
I took the morning off work and went to my first ever parent and child group today. I had been worried that it would be full of bored housewives gossiping but was pleasantly surprised that it was quite mixed and included among its number a big black male music producer who works mainly in Paris with a lot of groups Nolwenn had heard of. Indeed, I'd envisaged parents sitting around the edge of the room talking incessantly with cups of tea and digestives while the children played with, and fought over, a limited number of toys. I was actually impressed by the array of toys. What was really surprising to me was how busy all the mums were (and it was all mums apart from the big black guy and Nolwenn). They were rolling out play dough and cutting it into shapes, or assisting children

to paint, or passing bits of puzzle back and forth. No doubt if you interviewed them they'd say something about wanting to stimulate their children's mental development. I felt slightly aberrant ignoring Emile, who was quite happy whizzing about unsupervised, and talking to Nolwenn to practice my French – stimulating my own mental development in fact! At one point, all the little tables were pushed together and a little plate of fruit and nibbles served to the children. That's when the parents relaxed and had a good chat. After the children's snack came our tea and digestives and the session finished with us sitting in a circle for songs. I have attended my first playgroup – now I am proper mother!

Saturday 29th November 03.
Day 27 of my cycle. In the night I woke up feeling queasy (probably the amount of alcohol we drank while out) and felt a jolt of fear that I might be pregnant again.

Sunday 30th November 03.
As I lay in bed relaxing my first thought about being pregnant was that I hadn't taken folic acid this month. I'm becoming blasé it seems. I reach down and realise my period has started. No baby this month.
Eilish, still in pyjamas, hopped into my bed for a cuddle and then proceeded to tell me all the things she wants for Christmas: including one of those plastic domes that are full of water which when you shake them they look like it's a snow storm, vegetarian marshmallows, cake decorations (she'd spotted when we'd been out shopping), a new toy mobile phone, and a mirror. Six year olds are not too hard to please.
As the remote controlled racing car is now Emile's favourite toy I'm going to buy him a remote controlled duck I saw in the Early Learning Centre; I thought was quite funny. I've bought him more shape puzzles because he really likes them but I feel disinclined to buy more because he already has so much stuff. (Rumy, Robert's father, said that he'd never seen a baby with so many toys. And I imagine most of the people he knows in England are fairly wealthy).

Wednesday 3rd December 03.
I have been slumped in a slough of despond alternating with periods of

intense fury that my 'line manager', a term they prefer at my University to that of 'head of department', (just as, in the same way, they have a 'learning resources centre' instead of a 'library', and so forth) on learning that my funding bid was unsuccessful, has suggested that I "refocus my energies on teaching" and wants to scrap my working at home agreement. There's no link between the two things. I pointed out, vigorously, that I already carry a full teaching load in a compacted workweek and that I actually 'fund' some of my research time through overtime. At the moment I am so angry I cannot focus on my bloody research – I just want to commit murder. How can women with children manage when their bloody employers keep meddling with their remits all the time? I haven't had two years with the same routine since I started. I hadn't realised at the time but her changing my remit radically both before and after my maternity leave was completely illegal – discriminatory in fact. I wish I'd been better informed.

Thursday 4th December 03.
To cheer myself up, as Robert's just read the first 10,000 words of this diary and likes it, I thought I'd ring Virago to see if they'd be interested in publishing it. Now that they have mated with Time Warner I'm not sure what sort of crossbreed Virago has become. I still think of it as a nice little workers co-operative full of very enthusiastic, politically active, feminists (probably where this should actually be published). Virago have told me that should I send my book as an 'unsolicited manuscript' it will languish unread among the dusty piles. It will surface after an unspecified wait only to be examined by an underling with insufficient influence. I said I wasn't in a hurry and that I thought an editorial assistant could probably do a very good appraisal of the book; however, it was forcefully suggested that I find a literary agency. I really can't imagine having an agent.
Why don't I already have an agent? The answer is that I've always dealt with publishers directly and none before made having an agent a prerequisite of being taken seriously and I have tended to publish the sort of academic work that doesn't make much money, but is highly regarded by other academics. Oh God, I really don't want to find an agent…

Friday 5th December 03.
This is an important day as Nolwenn leaves today. I shall drive her to the station this afternoon. Sabrina, her, almost anorexic and rather lugubrious, replacement, arrived on Monday. (God knows what she thinks of me as I've been so preoccupied by work stuff this week and have probably been looking very serious). Nolwenn has been inducting her into our routines, so I am superfluous. I'd have liked to have spent more time with Nolwenn before she left, because I like her so much, but Sabrina has been keeping her entertained and so I've caught up with work and the row about work (my manager and I had a raised voices conversation yesterday but she has agreed to drop the idea of changing my working agreement for the time being; however, it [the threat of changing the agreement] remains a stick for her to beat me with whenever she chooses to get it out).

Saturday 6th December 03.
I had hoped to read in bed as a treat in the morning but ended up getting up as Sabrina needed to see a doctor and the doctor was only on duty until 10am. In the car on the way back I told her she was looking sad (she has had a face of thunder for days) and asked her what was wrong. She told me that her ex-boyfriend (of two months) had found a new girlfriend already. "If I was there", she proclaimed in her thick French accent, "I would kill them both". When expressed dismay at this idea she said replied, "well I would perhaps just beat them"...

Sunday 7th December 03.
I went to see a play, '*The Vagina Monologues*', with Robert last night. There weren't many other men in the audience; however, after a sketch about Brian, a man who loved vaginas, the actors thanked the men in the audience for coming and wondered if there were any Brians amongst them. A woman in the row behind us pointed at her husband and screeched, "He's a Brian, he's a Brian", which drew general applause. The play was composed of a mixture of one liners and monologue pieces. These were based on interviews with women who had been asked the question: if your vagina could talk what would it say? The reply, "SLOW DOWN" got the biggest laugh.

Tuesday 9th December 03.

We had our first trying-to-make-baby-sex of this month snuggled up under the duvet; it's freezing at the moment. It was leisurely and Robert made sure I had an orgasm though blew the mood later. After asking me about how I was feeling, he said, "so that means I can have a selfish fuck tomorrow".

I've seen a job I'm thinking of applying for and wonder how it would be being pregnant in a new job

Wednesday 10th December 03.

I didn't go swimming today, as I didn't want to risk flushing out Robert's sperms. (It doesn't bear thinking about what might be lurking in the water. But at least the chlorine would render it sterile…). Last night he was a very conscientious lover again, making sure I reached orgasm before he came himself.

Thursday 11th December 03.

At the bus stop was a woman with a hajib wound tightly around her head. I wouldn't have given her a second thought except that the end of the scarf was clenched firmly in her mouth and from time to time she chewed on it a little. I wondered if this was a common custom of her place of origin or a personal eccentricity. France has just outlawed the wearing of hajibs, along with other 'ostentatious' displays of religious affiliation in its schools. In the taxi, at the other end of my journey, the Muslim taxi driver was listening to the French minister for culture on the radio fielding telephone questions. The person phoning suggested that a child could remove her hajib as soon as she was through the school gates if she didn't want to wear it and therefore girls shouldn't be seen as forced to wear it; however, this didn't allow for the possibility that the child would be frightened that other children or the teacher might mention the lack of scarf to her fundamentalist parents. Anyway, I'm with the French on this one. I don't want to go any see "a play about Mary and Jesus" tomorrow (Eilish didn't push it fortunately, too distracted by her preparations for and of end-of-term disco was she).

Friday 12th December 03.

I didn't swim yesterday and I'm not swimming today. I know that pre-conception fitness is very important but I'm convinced that the chlorine in the pool damages the sperm (or at least it privileges the 'male' sperm, which is not what I'm wanting). I won't swim again until Tuesday (day 17 of my cycle). This would be the best time for me to get pregnant as my spring term is easier than my autumn term and I'd be heavily pregnant in the summer.

Sunday 14th December 03.

Robert jumped on top of me in the morning which means that we have managed sex from Tuesday (day 10 of my cycle) every day through to Sunday (day 15 of my cycle). Since my last two periods were 26 and then 28 days in length, I must be ovulating between day 12 and day 14. Come on sperm – you can do it!

To swim, or not to swim? We always do fortnightly and I didn't want to miss out, though on this occasion I could easily have opted out as Sabrina offered to join us. She said the water was too cold, and got out after 10 minutes, so it's just as well I was there as our water romps normally last at least two hours or so. Emile is getting quite confident at floating with his armbands on now and Eilish has now started diving and swimming under the water.

Monday 15th December 03.

Last night I put *Zadok The Priest* (Handel) on in Eilish's room as her homework was 'play a piece of music and identify as many different instruments as possible'. Before too long Eilish was cavorting all over the room doing a dance to the music and then Emile was copying her, which was absolutely hilarious. Robert came in and curtailed this frivolity, as inevitably he does. It's the price we pay for a well-regulated household.

Wednesday 17th December 03.

After working non-stop since Monday morning, I thought I'd do a little relaxing gift-wrapping. Three hours later I am exhausted from all the bending and stretching. Well exhausted is exaggerating but it's tiring. I haven't even started wrapping Emile's gifts yet. He has a Christmas party at his nursery at 2.30pm and I can't resist taking him round, even if I don't stay for the whole thing. Robert's going to put the tree up at the weekend. Eilish will help decorate it. Because it will get trashed in the children's play room and because there's no space for it in Robert's room, (which is full of wide-sceened TV, CDs and records, leather sofa and other male accoutrements…), it's going up in here where we'll have present opening on the day. I can't say I'm looking forward to living with the tree; kitch isn't really my thing.

In the afternoon, at the children's party, a troupe of nursery staff appeared in fancy dress, including a six foot tall black man in a snowman's outfit (slightly iconoclastic looking), a fairy, Father Christmas and an elf. Emile was actually quite freaked out. He didn't want to take the gift from Father Christmas when we visited the grotto, and indeed, he evinced no enthusiasm for the entire proceedings at all until he was offered a tangerine.

Robert thought my response to the idea of Father Christmas was hilarious. When we first met, when he asked me if I told Eilish that her presents came from Father Christmas I responded, that "I wasn't going to let a fictional patriarchal figure take the credit for all my hard work". I guess I was in slightly militant single parent mode at the time.

Thursday 18th December 03.

Today Eilish had a long awaited play session with Tom, a rather sweet and diminutive boy from her class. He was fine but Eilish was over-boisterous to the point of near injury. At one point she was doing ballet moves standing on Emile's tricycle and looked in imminent danger of falling on him. On another occasion, I found them both in my clothes cupboard hiding behind the clothes rail (and treading on the ends of my long dresses) at which point I got close to getting grumpy… Most of the time they spent "hiding from Emile" (in her play box, behind curtains, under the sofas). All in all, the experience was rather stressful. I'm glad that his parents had declined my invitation for him to stay to dinner.

The only thing that marred the day was Ian Huntley's imprisonment for the murder, and possible sexual assault, of two little girls, which dominated the news.

Friday 19th December 03.

It's a bitterly cold day. There was frost on the grass till mid morning. The sun seems to create some light but no warmth and despite having the central heating turned on full blast I feel cold as I sit at this desk.

Emile was ill today. After he'd been sick twice at the nursery they phoned Robert's mobile to ask him to come and collect him; however, he was stuck at the bus stop (for 85 minutes). When he phoned the transport information line to complain about the lack of buses, he was told that there was "grid-lock in the city centre". He came home in a foul mood. While he was cooking dinner, Emile, following two more vomits, lay on the couch and seemed too tired to raise his head to watch *Telly Tubbies.* Suddenly, he became really white and cold and I was momentarily paralysed by fear. My tears came gushing. I've been researching infant mortality and infanticide for an academic book I'm working on, but have been quite emotionally distanced from my subject matter, and I think at that moment it all became very real for me.

Following my sudden weeping fit, it occurred to me that I might have conceived, as being lachrymose was what characterised the onset of my last two pregnancies. The first was in St Petersburg, where I was attending a conference and being disorientated and far from those I love no doubt contributed to my breaking down. On my second night, snuggled up in bed, I sobbed myself to sleep. That was even before my period was late. I'd realised. I had actually told the friend I stayed with in London overnight, en-route to Russia, who kindly drove me to the airport, that I thought I was pregnant. It was just a peculiar hunch.

During my pregnancy with Emile, I got lost in London and couldn't work out where to get the train to the outer suburb where Robert was staying with friends. In the middle of a crowded station, having wasted what felt like an eternity of time trying to find the right platform, I suddenly found myself blinded by tears…

Anyway, with me feeling fragile and Robert in a bad mood, I guess it was inevitable that we should argue. We had friends to dinner: two film makers, and the evening went well. After the guests had gone, he was rude to me and sometimes that just makes me lose my temper. I wish I had more self-control, but sometimes I just lose it. I find rudeness, which indicates lack of respect, particularly provoking, because it reflects the dynamics that existed between my parents. My father, deeply unhappy, constantly insulted and belittled my mother who simply put up with it most of the time. Therefore, if Robert insults or depreciates me I can find myself overwhelmed with anger and shouting before I've even realised it has happened, and I suppose it is my father I'd like to annihilate (when I scream) for the way he treated my mother for so many years.

Saturday 20th December 03.
Maristella, a former au-pair, is visiting today and has just whisked off the children to the shops. Maristella, I think because she is older than most au-pairs who tend to be in their early twenties, is more like a trained nanny than an au-pair. She is buying new shoes for Eilish, having noticed that her school ones are getting a bit tight. (Eilish has just had a growing spurt and is much taller than most of the children in her class). Eilish is getting new boots for Christmas but Maristella is right, she does need new shoes. She's also buying new batteries for a remote-control toy Emile adores, because it conked out while they were playing with it. I'm sure if she were staying for a few days she'd sort out all the minutiae that needs attending to (all the stuff only I usually notice).
I did my last shopping and card sending yesterday and the traffic was wild and the shops packed so I'm glad to miss out on the final frenzy. At the cash machine yesterday there was such a huge queue I didn't want to wait for cash.
Well, Robert and I are about to sally forth in to a very wet evening. I guess everywhere will be heaving with people celebrating the last weekend before Xmas. He's been giving me the silent treatment all day so I'm wondering how the evening will go. During our nadir (tensions rose in October prior to the move) I actually flounced off twice when we out on Saturday nights as he was being so hostile and argumentative. Also, it's a year to the day since my miscarriage and I imagine that is also weighing on his mind. In bed last night I wondered what life would have been like had I had the baby and I realised we'd not be in this house. Even with Rumy's substantial bridging loan we couldn't have afforded it without my full-time salary (which would have been curtailed around now). Indeed, we'd be bracing ourselves for a year of financial hardship. Stuck with a newborn baby in Robert's semi, I wondered if I'd have been happy? I

imagine I'd have felt quite claustrophobic spending my year of maternity leave in that small space.
Anyway, I suspect we both wish to get into a peaceful frame of mind for Christmas. We have had an unprecedentedly peaceful and harmonious few weeks and have both been enjoying each other's company. So I think we both have that in mind. Furthermore, I do think I'm pregnant, though I'm not going to say anything. My period is due on the day after Boxing Day. Anyway, I can't face the thought of putting up the Christmas tree until Robert and I are being warm and loving to each other again, so I hope that happens soon.

Sunday 21st December 03.
Sabrina (our au-pair) is ill in bed with gastro-enteritis, which meant that Robert was sulking about having to look after Emile rather than have his normal four hours *Observer* newspaper gorge. I don't know why he wants another child if he can't just throw himself, with unbridled enthusiasm, into engaging with the ones we've got. We've had a tense day. This has included me updating my CV (not a fun task) and doing a huge Christmas supermarket shopping. Emile started trying to pull things off the shelf, saying "mine". In the end, I bought him a packet of rusks to keep him quiet.
I did let Robert put up the tree and then Eilish decorated it. She was in ecstasy and has done rather a good job, though it took about three hours. Or rather I should say, Robert bullied me into doing the tree because we'd agreed we'd put it up today, even though I said I'd prefer to wait a day, so that I could do it with unalloyed enthusiasm. My feelings seem to be irrelevant in this relationship. Likewise, he bullied me into doing the Christmas shopping – ditto I'd rather have left it a day or two.
At dinner Robert snapped at Eilish for asking an innocent question about whether she had been given the same as Emile (it was just a different bowl). Again, I wonder about his sanity… Often I think of Robert as being just mildly obsessive compulsive in a sort of harmless way but then I'm reminded that it impinges on, and damages, all of us. I don't want Eilish to become too timid to ask questions. I want to have relaxed mealtimes… I want us to have a happy Christmas but I think Robert is constitutionally incapable of being happy. He was snappy with me too but I placated him

rather than shouting back. Nevertheless, I went to bed in one of my dark *I've got to get out of this relationship* moods.

Monday 22nd December 03.
I spent my first free day applying for three jobs: two 'chairs' and a lecturing position. It was one of those very tedious sessions but now I've updated everything future applications, if necessary, should be much quicker. Sabrina came in and said she had to talk to me. Apparently, her boyfriend has asked her to come back. She wanted my opinion and I asked lots of questions such as: "Is he kind?" and "Is he faithful?" and "Does he take out his bad moods on you?" and "Is he honest?" as well as, "Do you think he's the man you'll have children with?", all questions to help her reflect on her situation. She is angry with him because he wanted her to abort their child, which she did, but she still weeps about it most days, she told me. Poor Sabrina, for a young person she has been through a lot: her step-father's suicide (only one year ago), the break-up with the boyfriend (with whom she was living), her mother's remarriage and move to an unfamiliar city, and weeping over her aborted baby.

Tuesday 23rd December 03.
I spent the morning paying bills, and doing necessary administration. When I mentioned this to Robert, he retorted that I'm incapable of relaxing. I explained that I want to do everything I need to do so that I can really relax and enjoy the fortnight's holiday. In the afternoon, I took Eilish swimming and we had a lovely time, including milk and cake in the café, which she loves. Now I feel like I'm on holiday at last!
During our French conversation practice session, I'd attempted to explain the origins of Zoroastrianism to Sabrina, and she'd seemed quite interested. I'd explained that it's a very ancient religion predating both Christianity and Islam; however, my French wasn't up to the challenge of talking about diaspora or suggesting that the Parsis are a bit like today's Jews of Europe (insular, professionally highly successful, discriminated against). Anyway, Emile began to demand attention, so the subject had to be dropped.
Over dinner, Sabrina asked Robert to tell her more about the Parsi religion. Robert replied that he wasn't interested in religion. I suggested

she ask Robert's father, who is coming for Christmas, and who is a practising Parsi, (hence why it had come up in conversation in the first place). Robert replied that if she raised the topic on Christmas day he'd end up "shouting" at his father! I hadn't realised his antipathy towards his father's culture was quite so entrenched (his mother is Swiss and blond, hence Robert's fair completion) but I should have foreseen this antipathy as he rejects anything Indian or religious. Even my buying Eilish a *Salwar-Chemise* to wear for the Parsi wedding feast before his sister's wedding had won no thanks. I even offered to wear a sari. "Why do Indians get to wear all the best clothes?", Eilish demanded once.

I was dreading his parents coming for Christmas but now anything that breaks the oppressive cloud, which is Robert's presence, is welcome, I feel. Perhaps, I just need more people around who will point out that Robert is unreasonable, bullish and rigid. That doesn't deal with the problem of his unreasonableness, bullishness and rigidity of course, but it might make me feel better!

Part of the reason I wasn't looking forward to their visit, (apart from Robert being ultra-tense for four days), is because Rumy only gives attention to Emile, in a way I find utterly offensive. I had assumed that it was because in Indian culture boys are everything and girls an inferior substitute, though I shouldn't generalise. Female infanticide and cultural norms, which regard girls as a contribution to the in-laws family and status (rather than the parent's own), are well documented. As I write this, I feel myself walking into a quagmire and want to back-out of it. Did I tell you that Robert's father is Indian (from Bombay)? We are a melting-pot family, an Irish, English, French, Swiss and Indian cocktail. Stir, and what do you get? The answer is – very pretty children.

Anyway, Robert recently suggested that Rumy's blatant favouritism isn't because he has misogynistic Indian ideas but because there is no blood link, which I think is even more offensive, or at least equally reprehensible, given that Robert is fathering Eilish. Emile doesn't look anything like Rumy anyway. I sometimes wonder what Rumy thinks of having a fair skinned, blue-eyed grandchild – perhaps I'll ask him if he's bothered that there is so little resemblance. His wife, Jacquie, is blond haired and blue eyed so obviously her genes and mine have stacked up against his, though if you look very carefully at Emile it's possible to see

slight shadowing under his eyes, so characteristic of Indians.
I digress, the other reason I'm dreading their visit is because Jacquie always manages to annoy Robert (or Rumy) by saying something gauche (not that Robert is by any means free of this affliction himself). I've seen him snap at her several times now. She is a native German speaker (a Swiss-German dialect) and learnt English in New York State, so has something of a North-American twang. Rumy and she met when she was nursing and he was a surgeon. She assisted him in performing grisly operations – "pass me the scalpel nurse Jacquie" – not a potentially romantic setting I would have thought. They discovered that they shared a love of classical music and it took off from their going to concerts together.
Anyway, no doubt there are thousands of people all round Britain who, at this very moment, are dreading the arrival of various relatives.

Wednesday 24th December 03.
Robert and I made love this morning. Well, it was more of a fuck, if I have to be honest about it. But the point is that we are being friendly. He has been very loving all day in little ways I appreciate. Also he's promised to take me out for a drink tonight, after the children are in bed, which I appreciate (he only likes going out on Saturdays usually).
Unfortunately, Eilish is ill. It's her turn to be sick. She's been looking very white and fragile, poor thing. She was only able to eat a little bit of bread for lunch.
Jacquie and Rumy arrived early afternoon and have brought mounds of things with them, including a very impressive home-baked cake which made Eilish's eyes light up. Jacquie has brought lots of treats including ginger bread and chocolate but we can risk her having any. They have all gone off to the botanical gardens leaving me in splendid peace.
My sister and family are due to arrive at 6pm laden with gifts and will demand a tour of the house, which they have not yet seen. We will then have six adults and four children here, which seems about right for a Christmas Eve in such a big house.
I feel absolutely certain I am pregnant. I wish I'd popped into *Boots* to get a pregnancy test. It would such a wonderful Christmas gift to give to Robert. The only little voice of doubt is because of the gastro-enteritis

going around, even though I've had my bout, I wonder if I'm still a bit ill, rather than pregnant…

Thursday 25th December 03.
Sabrina, who has decided to return to her boyfriend in France, is putting hair braids in Eilish's hair, and everyone else is watching junk television so I get this little opportunity to make an entry on the day itself. After a walk in the morning came the big feast and after that a marathon of present opening, which was almost too much, even for me. It was reasonably civilised with us all taking turns to open a gift and Eilish choosing them and handing them out to everyone. Emile's second birthday is on the 29th , so we put back a few of Eilish's gifts for her to open then when he opens his. Actually, Emile wasn't interested in opening things but he did like his *La La* telly-tubby and adored the remote controlled duck which goes round in circles as well as forwards and backwards, so it's a bit more complex than his racing car (yes, I do try to justify this excess to myself!). Robert exercised restraint; I know he wanted to say he found the whole thing repugnant but he managed to hold himself back. He is critical of materialism, except when it comes to his wide-screened TV, sound-systems (plural), huge record, CD, and book collections, tailor-made and designer clothes and so forth…

Friday 26th December 03.
Robert and I finished Christmas day by taking an evening walk. Exploring the local area, we found two local playgrounds we hadn't known about. On our return, I made the error of agreeing to watch some home video footage taken by Rumy which I found slightly irksome because of its obsessive focus on Emile and the voice-over, "now Emile is about the climb up the steps, he's sitting at the top of the slide, Emile is looking all around him…" and so on *ad-nauseum*. At one point I had to ask if Eilish had actually come on a particular trip, so out of the picture was she. Nevertheless, it was a successful day with no significant points of tension between us all. Rumy is actually a bit ill, with something he picked up during his flight from Miami, so has been less the genial patriarch than usual – which is a good thing.
Today, Boxing Day, after a few inevitable chores, we took the children to

a local park and I've just retuned from a walk with Robert, which ended in icy rain –exhilarating but not quite what I had in mind. Jacquie is making 'bugs' with Eilish in the kitchen. I can't hear Emile but I suppose he's up in the playroom with Sabrina or Rumy, but that reminds me to check in case no one had roused him from his afternoon nap. Tonight we are going to have a meal at a restaurant to give Robert a break. It looks as though we might achieve a row free Christmas.

Saturday 27th December 03.
My period started in the night. I felt sad. Time is running out and I am beginning to wonder if I'm actually capable of conceiving.

Sunday 28th December 03.
There were three pieces on maternity services in *The Observer* today – all saying roughly the same thing: that there is now a shortage of midwives. Secondly, that the transformation of birth into a high-tech 'medicalised procedure' is concurrent with the closure of community birth centres. The latter, run by midwives, are cost effective and offer continuity of care, so are important if birth is to be a 'rewarding' experience; however, they do not deal in medical emergencies so women experiencing these must be moved from community birth centres to obstetric units. One piece concluded that whilst, 'Hi-tech units and specialist support have saved many thousands of lives… we should not lose the wider picture. Childbirth is not an illness. It is the most natural event of all.'

Monday 29th December 03.
In the morning Sabrina announced that she felt "like the dead now living". I gave her the word 'resurrected'. One of my guests felt her behaviour was "inappropriate in front of the children", but I'm not sure what I can do. She is sitting for increasingly long periods with her head slumped in her hands and doesn't seem to eat anything. I am beginning to fear for the children's safety in her care. When I took her to the doctor she was told that she should seek medical treatment on her return to France. I wasn't impressed by that response.
Emile's birthday went well and he managed to blow out the candles on the cake. Eilish enjoyed helping him open his presents. At two, he's still too

young to be very excited by new things.

Tuesday 30th December 03.
I decided I should try to be firm. I told Sabrina that she must eat if she is to look after the children, otherwise she may faint and endanger their safety. In the morning she ate, literally, about ten pieces of cereal and I was left feeling very troubled. We have got bowls of fresh fruit, dried figs and dates, cupboards burgeoning with different foodstuffs… My guests discovered that Sabrina would eat Scottish shortcake – at last! Something apart from *Frosties* she says she enjoys – a miracle! Given that cooking is Robert's main hobby and great passion, and that he has a fantastic repertoire of haut cuisine, it's ironic that she will not eat anything he makes. At best, she has been eating bread and butter while we tuck into a rich array of Mediterranean or Indian dishes.

Sunday 4th January 04.
Today when we returned from swimming, Sabrina and her things were gone. She'd negotiated to leave on the 19th but obviously the lure of being back with her ex-boyfriend was too great and she was scared to tell us. Robert said he felt very relieved that she was gone. I felt anxious about interim childcare until our new au pair arrives, but I was also relieved, as her behaviour was getting very odd. I think she was suffering from manic depression as she was upbeat and lively occasionally and 'woe is me' the rest of the time – despite the reconciliation with her boyfriend.

Monday 5th January 04.
This morning, over breakfast, I tried to explain about the recent earthquake in Iran to Eilish. I showed her a picture of a weeping woman who had lost her entire extended family. Eilish burst into tears so I wish I hadn't. Perhaps she should be allowed to live in innocence for a little longer…
Today is an 'inset day'; a mysterious term employed by schools which means that the school is closed to pupils. (Fortunately, I'd booked the day as annual leave thinking Sabrina unable to cope with two children on her own). We have had Play Dough, Drawing, Telly Tubbies, and lunch, and now they are both in our back garden (which is walled and perfectly safe,

though I admit to peeking at them several times). They are decorating the walls with chalk drawings, or scribbles in Emile's case, at present. Eilish has been instructed to inform me immediately if Emile starts uprooting shrubs! It's almost time for his nap at which time I'll put Eilish in front of cable TV so I can get to read for an hour. I've discovered a channel which seems quite suitable, called *Cebeebies*.

The local nursery, which Emile has been attending twice a week, has a full-time place for him until the new au-pair arrives which is very very lucky.

Tuesday 6th January 04.

Today my morning started in a lovely way with my dressing my little 'tuppy' and giving his breakfast. He's so cuddly and gentle in the mornings. He wakes up smiling. "Where's Elilish?" he asks perkily. I don't think he understands my reply. Clearly, he has the correct attitude to life - or the correct cocktail of chemicals swishing around in his petite metabolism. When I left him at the nursery he didn't cry.

At work I had a tutorial, and as the student came into my room I heard myself invite her: " do climb in over the piles of unmarked essays" which were virtually covering my office floor. I saw myself then in my work persona: slightly dishevelled after the long drive to work, sitting in a shambolic and seedy looking office, my long blond hair tied up in an unflattering bun, literally surrounded by piles and piles of work and with 143 unread e-mails in my virtual in-tray. If anyone thinks being an academic is glamorous they should think again. I never get to finish it all, never…

Wednesday 7th January 04.

It's day 12 of my fertility cycle so guaranteed sex tonight. Sex today to Saturday inclusive and I'll have my last swim this afternoon, as I don't want to disadvantage the 'female' sperm with chlorine.

On Women's Hour this morning various women were debating the pros and cons of having children early or late in life. Some thought older women were more patient and more emotionally capable of dealing with the challenges of dealing with young children. Others felt that older mothers would be more boring, though an older mother, brought on for comment, vigorously refuted this. Having done lots of "going out and travelling" in her youth one older mother explained she didn't resent having to stay in a lot (the implication being that had she been a younger mum she might have resented it). Personally, when I was younger I lacked the courage, initiative and money to do many of the things I'd now like to do, so that doesn't really hold for me.

Another woman said she'd have liked a larger family but at 43 (my age, almost) she didn't want to try because of the increased risks. Although intellectually I know that when I have CVS I may be told that my child has Spina-Bifida, or some other terribly debility, I haven't given any thought as to how I might deal with it.

My big regret, if I have one, is that I didn't simply sign myself off sick when I felt ill with my last pregnancy, the one that miscarried. Why did I carry on slogging away? Why? And for an institution which shows so little appreciation. Why did I sacrifice my baby for a bloody university?

Well, I better get down to some marking. They are still paying my wages.

Thursday 8th January 04.

Even though sex is guaranteed, or so I thought in my ovulation period, I'd made an effort last night, doing my hair how he likes it, wearing lipstick (his big fetish), his favourite briefs (his other fetish: they have to be a certain sort of material), having moisturised my skin, shaved my legs and applied lavish amounts of perfume after my shower.

Robert couldn't get an erection. Well, I should say he had one but he lost it. We spent ages kissing, caressing each other and I ended up sucking his flaccid dick to no avail. I was left feeling tearful and humiliated. I lay in the dark thinking that I'm never going to have another baby…

Friday 9th Janauary 04.

I made even more effort last night adding lingerie to the list of things I know pleases him. While he was in the shower, I looked at myself in full-length mirror in our bedroom. I may be forty-two but I looked HOT. Lots of men would like to fuck me so how did I end up with someone so lacking in libido?

Robert explained that he'd had wind, which had made him feel "unsexy", and that lack of erection had "nothing to do with me". As the woman who'd had a flaccid dick in her mouth on Wednesday night, I couldn't quite see it like that, but felt reasonably reassured.

Robert and I kissed for a while and then he got a big erection and for some reason wanted me to suck him. He knelt over me in a dominating manner while I licked his dick, but the erection disappeared again. He announced that he felt under "too much pressure". He asked me not to be angry. He let me sit on his face for a while (it happened spontaneously as we were sucking each other with me on top, in a final attempt to get him erect) but, unusually, I couldn't get close to orgasm because he'd spoilt my mood. Also, I can tell when he's really enjoying sucking me and when he's not totally involved in it, and it felt as though he was trying to pleasure me from guilt – though I might be wrong.

This is one problem I simply hadn't foreseen. Robert had had difficulty getting erections with his ex (whom he had ceased to fancy) but never with me. I know he does find me sexually attractive, well at least if I do all the thing he likes, so that's not the problem. I guess it is the pressure. But what are we to do?

All I could think of to propose is that we have sex before the optimal days so that if we miss day 12 and 13, as we did have this month, at least we'd know I was full of sperm anyway so might conceive anyway. I suggested that this might take the pressure off for the most likely days, which are twelve to fourteen. He said he thought he'd feel under pressure anyway because it would still be about conception. Seeing he was upset I didn't think it was worth trying to reason with him. I imagine it's brought back his nightmares from his previous relationship which I had hoped were forgotten.

At my age, I can't afford to miss an ovulation. Today is day 14, probably the last day I can possibly conceive in this month's cycle. Will he manage an erection tonight?

Saturday 10th January 04.

Robert was positively self-congratulatory after managing to get and sustain an erection last night. He whizzed off and got a glass of brandy to toast "your orgasm, filling you with seed, and my erection".

I must admit I wasn't even expecting us to attempt sex. When he came into the bedroom I was engrossed in *The Fruit Expert*, and planning what sort of trees to plant and where in the garden. I expected us to just cuddle. But he heaved me out of bed and we stood and looked at each other and kissed and before long he was erect. I couldn't just relax and enjoy it though, as any second I was expecting him to deflate but, perhaps out of guilt, he was particularly tenacious and waited for my orgasm before he groaned out his load.

As we have no au-pair at present, this two hours during Emile's nap will be the only time I get to write at the weekends. Even our usual babysitters are busy so we are going *en famille* to Pizza Express tonight with the children, rather than staying in. I imagine Emile will refuse to sit in his high chair. He's very frisky at the moment and doesn't like sitting still at all. The good thing is that it's only a ten minute walk away so at least it will be easy to get home if it all goes disastrously wrong and we have to bolt when he starts annoying other customers…

Sunday 11th January 03.

Well, Robert gave last night's Pizza Express outing nine-and-a-half out of ten, though he thought his pizza was bland. Both children were immensely well behaved, except for Emile at the beginning who threw various things of the floor, including his knife and fork. Fortunately, it's quite noisy there so the utensils clattering to the ground didn't cause him to become the centre of attention. There was a pianist I thought would amuse Emile while we waited for the food but he didn't seem very interested. Perhaps he's too used to seeing his grandfather play for it to be a novelty.

My pizza was quite good and the wine was fine and Eilish was in heaven when we had ice cream for dessert. Later, when we slumped into bed neither of us had the energy for sex though.

We are about to head off to the swimming pool now. Both children adore swimming so it's always a pleasure to take them.

***

The Observer had one of those thoroughly depressing articles about how it's impossible to have a career and be a mother. It stated the following cheerful facts:

An average of three women per day register claims of pregnancy-related unfair dismissal.

That there is a 20% difference between the hourly salaries of men and

women working full-time.
That only 2% of executives in the FTSE top 100 companies are women.
That only 18% of MPs are women.
More than half of all women have experienced some sort of sexual harassment at work.

Monday 12th January 03.
Robert and I had a massive row last night and I lost my temper when he was sneering at me. That's right sneering at me: "you're pathetic". It was the way he was drawling out the words which made me snap. He's taking the high-moral ground though because I'm the one that shouted. That's a joke isn't it? It's my problem and I'm the one that must apologise because I ended up making more noise. His emotional violence, because it's quieter, doesn't count. I've told him we must go to RELATE. I'm sick of his aggression every time I try to express any feelings or opinions.

Tuesday 13th January 03.
Elodie has confirmed she can come to join our family at the weekend. A new au-pair to induct is always a lot of work, but having no au-pair is a lot of work too. I miss never having lay-ins more than anything, as I have to give Emile his breakfast and take him the nursery in the mornings. I crave being able to lie in bed for as long as I need.

Wednesday 14th January 03.
I was feeling really really tired before Christmas so I went to see my G.P. who said I should have some blood tests which I had last week. Robert knew the results were due yesterday but he hasn't asked me about them. It's not my paranoia that he doesn't care about me. He really doesn't care about me. I'm not sure I should have a baby with this man. Row, or no row, his not asking is unforgivable.

Saturday 17th January 04.
Elodie arrived chaperoned by her father, Marc. We immediately both liked her and he was an absolute charmer of about my age. He has quit his business job and is doing lots of acting and script writing – finding himself in 'mid-life' I suppose, following his separation from Elodie's mother.

Saturday 18th January 04.
Robert announced this morning that he is over our last row. He has been sulking all week, though the arrival, on Wednesday, of a large quantity of late Christmas presents from my ex-husband's family didn't help his mood at all. I told Mary (my ex-husband's mother), and put it in writing to her, that Eilish wasn't coming to visit during this holiday because we had guests who wanted to see Eilish but she's suffering from poor memory now so hence the late gifts... Indeed, she'd rung me a few days ago to find out when Eilish was coming and had an absolute tantrum when she discovered she wasn't.
On Saturday night, Robert admitted feeling upset. He had thought that my ex living in Australia would mean never have to deal with all this – the fact of there being another family. He hadn't realised that the Douglas family are all rather fond of Eilish and want to maintain some sort of relationship with her, though Mary has been too busy picking up honorary degrees and giving lectures at Yale to give Eilish a second thought until a lull arose in her busy schedule. Then, when I didn't respond exactly as she wished to her clicking her fingers she didn't like it. The rest of the family are acting out of a Catholic sense of duty – I don't feel that any of them know or love her.
I am thinking angry thoughts: I don't have sympathy for any of them. I never agreed to lie to Eilish about her parentage. Robert's assumption, that because the progenitor was indifferent the entire extended family would be too, was unrealistic. I don't feel at all comfortable about the idea of pretending to Eilish that Robert is her biological father – the fact that he's doing the day-to-day parenting is the meaningful thing – surely? He ***is*** her father. He is the only one she's ever had; but I won't lie to her.
Furthermore, I am not prepared to cut off the Douglas's, as Robert would wish. On the other hand, Mary has been too bloody self-obsessed to form a relationship with her granddaughter so I think she has forfeited, though her own behaviour, much consideration on my part. I don't feel guilty for not putting myself out for her on this occasion. Anyway, the whole thing's an absolute emotional quagmire.

***

The Observer Magazine had an article in it called *Mother's Ruin*, highlighting that 10% of maternal deaths (deaths within one year of the birth) are caused by suicide. The epicendocrine changes following childbirth were described as 'unmatched' by any other biological event. Indeed, the body's craving for steroid hormones, such as cortisol, oestrogen and progesterone were likened to withdrawal effects experienced in giving up alcohol or heroin. Yes, we become hormone junkies and some of us overcome our pregnancy addictions better than others. I poor myself a glass of brandy and congratulate my body on overcoming all my hormone dependency… just joking.

Monday 19th January 04.
I discovered I am not short-listed for a professorial job I was actually invited to apply for. I feel humiliated.

Tuesday 20th January 04.
I catch the headline of a tabloid newspaper on my way home as I stop to fill up with petrol, 'baby killers to be released'. I don't want to waste any time going back to buy a copy as I've already paid for my petrol when I notice it. Later, the radio tells me that it's a review of prosecutions which were based on symptomatology called 'shaken baby syndrome', which has now been discredited. But I am rushing home to be with Emile knowing that Eilish will already be asleep after I have worked another exceptionally long day in the office (8am to 7.30pm). I feel so sad that work impinges so much on my home life and can think of nothing else, as I drive through the dark, than the lovely feeling of holding my baby and stroking his gorgeous soft, sweet smelling, hair and breathing him in.

Wednesday 21st January 04.
Our new au-pair, Elodie, has *mal du pays,* otherwise known as home sickness. She burst into tears over breakfast so, even though I have a pile of urgent cross-marking to do, I spent the morning trying to cheer her up. I was in a very in a cheerful mood, fortunately. We all went to see the Winter Garden (a big modern glass dome filled with tropical plants) and the shops and I got Elodie registered at the library and also at my health club (as a welcome gift I have given her a month's membership). She then got a tour of the facilities at the club which wet her appetite, I hope. After that, I took her to the post-office to get stamps for France. Then, when

Emile went to the nursery in the afternoon she went shopping and I hunkered down to do my marking.

Thursday 22 January 04.

I have a very upset stomach today but I did manage a walk in the botanical gardens first thing in the morning with Elodie and Emile which was refreshing. Today is day 27 of my cycle. At this time every month I am filled with expectation. If my period has not arrived by Sunday I am probably pregnant.

I am sorting out some papers, Emile's birth certificate for place of birth says: 'Bramall Lane Roundabout, Sheffield on the way to The Jessop Wing, Royal Hallamshire Hospital, Sheffield.'

Friday 23 January 04.

I took Elodie and Emile to the local parent and child group in the morning and she seemed to enjoy it. There was a woman just arrived from India, called Kavitha, who gave us her telephone number so that we can meet at the local park – that will be nice for Elodie, who doesn't like being alone, and it will be nice for Kavitha, who has only been here a week and who doesn't know anyone.

My period started yesterday evening… There were a lot of babies at the group and it made me feel sad.

Saturday 24 January 04.

I almost forgot to mention that my *Sex and the City* is back on screen, with an episode entitled *'Let There be Light'*. Ever wondered why you feel emotionally vulnerable after sex? It's all down to hormones released during intercourse according to Carrie Bradshaw, who suggests that women's desire to bond is chemical.

Charlotte is wondering whether it's unfair on a potential employer to take a job when she's intending to start trying for a baby again (she had a miscarriage in the last series). I'd like to point out to her, as one who now knows, that conception can take a long time; however, I know how she feels. I'm thinking of applying for a new job but I know that if I have to write and deliver new lecturing material whilst pregnant I'll just be an exhausted wreck and a crap lecturer too! I think women shouldn't be obliged to work through their pregnancies at all. It's sheer cruelty. Indeed, women should be offered optional leave from the moment of conception.

Sunday 25th January 04.
There was a heart-rending piece in *The Observer Magazine* today on what happened to a girl born 16 weeks prematurely in 1996, who was fragile and sick for a long time even after she was over the worst: the worst being open-heart surgery, an operation to prevent blindness, and life threatening bouts of pneumonia. She also had a blood clot in her left hand, which caused it to go black, and it was almost amputated. Her early life at home entailed being on oxygen 24 hours a day and hooked up to a monitor. She couldn't cry for food because her voice box had been damaged by the ventilation tubes. Sometimes her nose would block up and she'd turn blue. She was also very vulnerable to infection so her mother hardly ever risked taking her out for the first 18 months, describing herself as "virtually housebound".
We are told that around £100,000 worth of equipment kept Sophie alive. It's a terrible ethical dilemma to spend such huge amounts on very premature babies when they often die or end up living with horrendous disabilities. We all have these images in our minds of these cute fragile little babies in incubators but in saving such babies earlier and earlier through the use of Caesarean Section we are inflicting upon the survivors a poor quality of existence and tremendous trauma for the parents.
This particular article is upbeat. The mother and daughter are happy and Sophie's disabilities are not emphasised in the article but include almost complete deafness, difficulty in eating, chronic lung disease and a general proclivity to sickness and tiredness. In the photo she smiles at the camera. She, it seems, is one of the luckier ones…

Monday 2nd February 04.
I sent a letter to my former mother-in-law to explain my current situation and to say, frankly, how I feel about her lack of interest in Eilish and her recent tantrum.

Tuesday 3rd February 04.
My life is running away with me again. It's their homework, the children's

need for attention, as well as the practical things, like remembering to check their hair for nits. My job is the biggest time-eater and I feel like a hamster in a little wheel. I rush from one thing to the next the whole time. I teach, mark, give tutorials, and fill in the endless forms: marking pro-formas, module evaluation reports, cross-marking assessments, photocopying requisitions, materials requests. I rush off in my lunch break to *Paks Foods* and stock up on fruit and vegetables. Then I write and photocopy student handouts, answer e-mails, talk to prospective students, and so forth, until it's time to introduce the guest lecturer. I listen attentively to the lecture so I can facilitate questions. Whatever I do, there is no respite and I never feel that I am quite on top of the job. Should I get a spare moment, there's that funding bid I haven't had time to look at or that Ph.D. application languishing… or my book (the academic one) that I never seem to get around to working on.

On Tuesday evenings I host a guest lecturing series for our post-graduate students. I suppose I'm identified with being an academic, last night's guest speaker said, "So you're a Reader", wanting to draw me out about my research interests, and I quipped that I don't get enough time to read; but I wasn't joking.

Emile has bitten Eilish in the face and she has a nasty bite mark as testament to his ferocity so I must break off my writing and go to her. (Our melancholy au-pair, Elodie, is sweet but not terribly efficient).

Wednesday 4th February 04.

I can hear the theme tune from the *Telly Tubbies* wafting from the playroom upstairs. Robert and I almost didn't have sex last night because we almost rowed. He is letting them watch totally inappropriate adult television on Mondays when I'm away, having previously agreed that on school days they should only see videos and that Children's TV would be a weekend treat. When I asked him to stop letting them watch the programmes in question he refused. I'd already told Eilish that she can't watch TV on Mondays so I pointed out that if he continues to let her watch it he is undermining my parental authority. Even this line of argument, aimed at his authoritarian streak, didn't work. I argued that the programmes have disturbing content and he retorted, "Look you're getting hysterical now". This is the sort of trigger remark that would have had me explode with anger in the past but I seem to be getting inured to his abusiveness, or able to exercise more adult self-control – depending on your perspective. I went off to calm down feeling very negative about him but, after I'd given the children their bath and done Eilish's reading practice and the bed time stories, we had a nice time cuddling Emile together and I was reminded how nice it is to be with him. Are relationships always THIS HARD?

Anyway, we did end up having sex. One Sunday night we'd had sex at bedtime and then again in the morning so "I'd be full of seed" for day 12 of my fertility cycle. So I guess if we have sex again tonight we'll have managed to get all my fertile days again, or what we now think are the peak days.

Thursday 5th February 04.

When I got home tonight at 7.30pm Emile heard my voice and climbed out his bath. He stood naked and cherubic at the top of the stairs. He's really so beautiful with his uncut curly hair and blue eyes. Then carefully he climbed down to greet me, eventually throwing himself into my arms. Only other parents can fully realise how wonderful such greetings are...

It's day 15 of my cycle so I imagine I've already conceived if I'm going to this cycle but we'll be having sex again tonight just in case.

Last night we had sex and then he jumped on me again this morning and was really big and hard until the alarm clock went off and then he just deflated... He's obviously feeling determined to impregnate me. I've enjoyed the sex this week but now I'd be quite happy to have a night off!

Friday 6th February 04.

It turns out Robert was too knackered to make love to me last night. Actually he did get an erection as we stood caressing each other but then he had wind again and this put him off (whatever will he be like by the time he is my age – quite wrecked I'm sure!). But the whole thing wasn't a disaster – he just looked at me and asked, "shall we cuddle?" and it was nice until Robert was unconscious – he just konks out. Laying in the candle-light was relaxing for a while but then I leapt out of bed and came down to my study to read. I wish I didn't dislike this room so much. Perhaps it's just the terracotta walls that are off-putting to me; however, the original early Victorian fire surround is positively funereal – I just can't look at it without thinking of graves – and the circa 1930s copper and turquoise tiled inset looks utterly incongruous. Furthermore, the shape of the room is long and thin with only one window. I don't want to seem ungrateful; a lot of people would adore this house; but I don't.

Some one else who is discontent in this house is Elodie, our new au-pair. As a friendly gesture, I went with her to the parent and baby group in the morning and she sat with her arms crossed looking so sour faced that none of the other parents spoke to her. Indeed, after about twenty minutes of attempting conversation with her, I decided to go and chat with other mums! She is always going to be socially isolated if she exudes misery… (Never hire an au-pair who has a boy friend back at home). I had a nice time playing with Emile and chatting. I was impressed that he did the actions for *Wind the Bobbin Up*, at song time. It's wonderful watching babies acquire new words and skills on a daily basis.

At first I thought she was just home-sick, but now I wonder if Elodie has some sort of bio-polar disorder, as she was sniffling whilst doing some housework after the group; however, by the evening she was chatting in an animated way on the phone… On Wednesday she was howling so loudly it disturbed me when I was trying to work at my desk. It affects my mood too having this miserable person in the house… I have predicted that she will resign after her boyfriend's forthcoming visit for St Valentine's Day; however, if she doesn't we will have to think about asking her to leave. She lacks enthusiasm for the children, which is a big negative, and never seems to remember to do the odds and ends she's supposed to do around the house. She'll sit looking bored, and it makes me feel like saying, well, "up we get, now, look at this basket of children's clothes which needs folding and putting away… no need to sit looking bored when there's so much that needs doing…" And indeed, I do remind her to do things but the next day they remain undone again, which is putting me in the tedious position of having to ask her to do everything she is supposed to do. I must e-mail her father to express my concern.

Anyway, I have got other things on my mind. I want to get chapter two of my new book started. And Robert and I had a G.P. appointment with Emile to discuss his undescended testicle. She suggested he may have to have surgery because the ball can become malignant if left to its own devices.

I can't bear the thought of my little baby having to undergo an operation… I don't know what the risks are attached to such surgery – general anaesthetic carries some risks. I'm sure Emile would rather have one ball than die! We are now on the waiting list to have a chat with a paediatric surgeon.

Saturday 7th February 04.

Maristella, our former au-pair (now studying at university in Scotland), has whisked the children off to a museum so I have this little bit of unexpected free-time. I should do some work on my new book; however, I picked up *The Guardian* Weekend and read a rather silly piece by Julie Bindel instead, in which she suggests that parents get 'more validation, support and access to public resources' that those who don't have children. As a working single parent with my first child, I discovered how little support there really is. There are no free nursery places for babies and the average nursery bill is £150.00 plus per week. This is not tax deductible. When I phoned *Surestart*, feeling absolutely exhausted, I was told that the volunteers only give social support not respite child care – which is what I was hoping for – just an hour or two off during a long winter's evening or weekend, or when I was ill, so I could get some bed-rest. My mother, who might have given me 'validation', was long dead. What resources? What support? What validation? None was forthcoming from the State. I guess it's easy for the childless to fantasise about what motherhood is like, but let's acknowledge that it is fantasy… Yes, I did get support and validation – but from other single mothers! My children are by far the most wonderful part of my life but I could have done with much more help in the beginning.

Furthermore, what about the opposite of 'validation' new mothers get from their childless friends – "you're not going to become a vegetable are you?" friends ask in subtle or less subtle ways. For example, "you are going to continue to write aren't you?" is a frequent one I get which translates as "Oh dear, she's going to become boring now." And what about that management role I was steered away from… surely I wouldn't do a good job with a new born? And would I mention that I am hoping to have another baby at interview for a new job? Absolutely, delighted to get the validation…

Sunday 15th February 04.

I am either ill or pregnant but have to wait until Wednesday, when my period is due, to find out. I suspect it was just something I ate.

Yesterday I was forty-three. I had an action packed day. I went to an acting workshop during the day and was offered a bit part in *Twelfth Night.* Robert was very disdainful as he loathes amateur dramatics and it would mean my being out for another evening each week for rehearsals. I pointed out that I am only out once per week for my own pleasure (I also teach on a Monday night and sometimes on a Tuesday too). I think it would be fascinating to be in the play. Still, it's hard to do something when ones partner is so down on it. I wish I could develop some immunity to his prejudices and opinions.

I played with the children for a couple of hours before going out to the theatre with Robert to see a really good performance of Arthur Miller's *The Crucible.* I'd seen it when I was younger but found it so much more poignant this time, twenty years later.

There was a very encouraging piece in *The Observer* about a new study, which has found a link between the age of the mother and the cognitive development of children. It seems that the children of older mums do 'significantly' better than those of younger mums. This isn't surprising really; with a Ph.D. under my belt and lots of life-experience I have far more to offer than when I was twenty – I'm just talking for myself you understand. The Study by Dr Julia Berryman of Leicester University looked at mothers over the age of thirty-five. Still, if Eilish has children as late as I did I'll be seventy-three by the time I have my first grand-child, a rather shocking thought… Will I still be able to be useful then? I don't want her children to see me as a slightly frightening, haggard, demented, old crone…

Monday 16th February 04.

In *Sex and the City* maternal themes predominate. Samantha loses her cool when, following her mastectomy, her doctor has the temerity to report the fact that childless women are more at risk of breast cancer than those who have suckled. She feels she is being "punished" for not having had children and has an irrational outburst suggesting that her doctor regards her as a "whore" who "deserves" to get cancer. It's weird fit of paranoia but as it was on mainstream television perhaps deserves mention.

Meanwhile, Miranda gives her baby son, Bradie, over to Carrie and Charlotte so she can take a long-weekend honeymoon. Needless to say, this gets the girls talking about motherhood. Carrie discovers that her boyfriend, Alexander, is great with Bradie. She visits him in his luxurious apartment with the baby. Bradie breaks a vase within seconds of their arrival. As Carrie fusses over the burglar alarm over it goes, and then in breezes Alexander who instantly calms the scene with a quip about Carrie being pathetic for blaming the broken vase on the baby. In the next scene we see Bradie painting and Alexander joking about his evident talent. Alexander is good with children – in all things North American the point has to be laboriously spelt out: "you're good with children", or something equally superfluous, spouts Carrie smilingly, bimbo style. Something stirs – could it be maternal instinct? Momentarily, she has the vision of him as the father of their child. Could it be? The romantic vision is shattered almost at once as she discovers that he has had a child and a vasectomy. She plucks up courage to talk to him: "vasectomies are reversible aren't they", she asks? "Not for me", he makes clear. She has allowed herself to fall in love with a man who has already lived that part of his life. She is thirty-eight; when is she planning on having a child, he asks? They are on a precipice. The show is developing an edge it didn't have before.

Charlotte who, we may recall, has recently had a miscarriage, thinks she should ditch the man rather than miss out on being a mother. Carrie is uncertain: "Why should I give up a man for a baby I hardly know I want", she asks herself? On the other hand, will Alexander love her enough to make-up for her not having a baby? It's too early in the relationship to be sure of that. He says if having a child is something she really wants she must have it: he will understand that she may wish to choose to leave him. Samantha encourages her to think, in a positive way, about what she'll have (or possibly have) if she chooses to remain childless.

In the soap *Friends,* Phoebe's brother turns up with his triplets and announces that he hasn't slept in three years! Phoebe says she'll take one of them off his hands but when he looks at each of them (they are dozing on a couch in the café where much of each episode is located) he can't bear the thought of parting with any of them. It was a crummy joke but I found it poignant because during Robert's and my nadir, which wasn't that long ago, I did think seriously about the possibility of taking off with Eilish and leaving Emile. I could relocate. I could cope. I'd be able to start a new life with just one child in tow – perhaps back in Australia where I used to live. But of course, I could not bear the thought of leaving him and when I imagined being without him I just felt bleak… No, it would destroy me to lose him, I realised.

Being in a new relationship wouldn't be a *raison de être* if I left Robert, but with two children in tow, from two different men, I imagine my eligibility in the marriage market would be somewhat diminished…

Tuesday 17th February 2004.

My period started two days early. I wonder if my menstrual cycle has always been this erratic. Perhaps I am very near to the menopause now.

Saturday 21st February 2004.

This morning Robert came back from shopping at 11ish to find Eilish and I eating half a slice of toast each. Perfectly normal you might think for a Saturday morning? But Robert was scowling at us through the window as though we'd committed a heinous crime. He'd intended to give us all an extra early lunch but he hadn't articulated this nor left a note. He was in a genuinely bad mood about it. I quipped that my psychic powers weren't switched on first thing in the morning. I also pointed out that half a slice of toast wouldn't spoil our appetite for an early lunch. Nevertheless, he was in a depressed, terse, mood for the rest of the morning.

The incident has had a very oppressive effect on my mood, reminding me that Robert is more than just a control freak; he genuinely has some sort of mild form of metal illness, which means that he simply cannot cope with things not happening in precisely the way that he envisaged. No matter how trivial, anything untoward spoils his mood. I thought he was getting more relaxed but this incident reminds me that he's seemed easier going *because he's been getting his own way all the time.* I just concede to him more than I used to. He suggests a schedule for the day and I go along with it. Some of his quirks I've just got used to. If I go to kiss him he shies away from me, for example. I don't mean snogging, I mean a peck on the lips. He shies away from me! Gratuitous kissing, it disturbs him; it's too spontaneous. I'm going to insist he goes to see a therapist. I know it will cause a row but I think he had to work on this obsessive-compulsive disorder of his. Does your husband have quirks like this I wonder?

Sunday 22nd February 04.
In '*Out of the Frying Pan into the Fire'* (this week's *Sex and the City*) Charlotte, who, the voice-over tells us, was good at everything at high-school and won all the prizes, isn't winning the 'baby-race'. Her partner checks out adoption and Charlotte tries to come to terms with the fact that it might not happen. She also acquires a dog!
In bed, I managed to tell Robert that I think he should see a therapist. It didn't cause a row but I don't think he realised that I am absolutely serious (I do joke a lot).

Monday 23rd February 04.
Fair's fair, I had my first psychotherapy appointment today. My therapist, a genial man of about my own age, thinks that the "annihilating rage" I express towards Robert, when I do lose my temper with him, is leftover anger towards my father for the way he treated my mother. This is probably true. I feel bored at the prospect of raking over all this stuff again.
The only time I felt raw emotion is when I talked about my *desire* to have another baby. Although in December 2002 I felt real relief when I had my miscarriage, as well as grief, I feel really ready now to have another baby. I feel physically and mentally well prepared. I feel that my body has had enough time to rest since the last birth. *I want a baby now – give me a baby* I am screaming inside.

Wednesday 25th February 04.
It's precisely one year since I started trying to have a baby. Like Charlotte, I don't like being a failure at something that is supposed to be *effortless* and *natural.*

Thursday 26th February 04.
I didn't go to the acting group tonight. I'd been wondering whether or not to go after Robert's negative response to the idea; however, a heavy

snowfall made a decision unnecessary, as it would have been impossible to drive to the venue except in a four-wheel drive vehicle with snow chains, which I don't have. I drive a miniscule Fiat: a motorised buggy in effect.

Day 10 of my fertility cycle and more baby-making sex is on our agenda for the next few days. I didn't even get out of bed after we'd made love so that I wouldn't lose any sperm. I let Robert blow out the candle and fetch my alarm clock. Since we'd both really like a girl the preconception sex is a good idea, because of the 'female' sperm's greater longevity.

Friday 27th February 04.

We've decided that we'll have sex tomorrow and on Sunday but we'll pause tonight. Actually, as soon as I write this I wonder if that's a good idea. Robert is reading me the complete works of Shakespeare in bed and is keen to finish off *Titus Andronicus* – a bloody conclusion is in store… This is the 'up side' of Robert's obsessive compulsiveness. He is reading all the critical literature he can find on each play; then he discourses upon it for my edification: explaining critical opinion, complex twists of plot or difficult words, before reading it to me. He reads very well. It's all rather enjoyable.

Today, because of the snow, Eilish is not at school because it's shut. She's upstairs tidying her room but I'm about to supervise her writing out her party invitations. I am beginning to despair of getting some research done.

Wednesday 5th March 04.

I announced confidently that I am pregnant. Robert pointed out that I said this before and was wrong. But then he asked me how I know and I quipped that it's just feminine intuition.

Thursday 6th March 04.

Today I had my meeting with the head of personnel to discuss my opting for a part-time contract. It's quite straightforward. I also got a clarification on parental leave. I'm due parental leave too now the E.C. regulations have come into force; however, my employer will only allow 4 weeks per child per year to be taken and they can postpone the date for commencement for up to six months. When I pointed out that it would be impossible to take the 13 weeks per child to which I am notionally entitled because of their 'implementation policy', she was adamant that the University is acting legally – even thought this will prevent me taking the full 26 weeks due. I imagine that many people who would most benefit from this legislation couldn't afford to take unpaid leave anyway…

I do wonder about writing this diary at a time when it's only really fashionable to come out as detesting motherhood. All I the books I've read recently about becoming a new mother have been angst ridden and none of the authors seemed about to simple relax and enjoy the experience. I like being a mother. Yes, I have moments of ambivalence, mainly stimulated by a feeling not having enough time to myself to read and write and relax, but I love being a mother. *I love being a mother.* Being with my children and enjoying them feels more meaningful *than anything else.*

***

Anyway, on quite a different tack, there's some good news for those women who were wrongfully imprisoned after being accused of smothering or shaking their babies to death. Following the successful case of Angela Cannings in December, whose appeal court judgement quashed her conviction for murdering two of her babies, a more open attitude is being taken to multiple baby deaths, which may be caused by viral illnesses which kill because of genetic weaknesses which have yet to be fully explained. The court of appeal called for a halt to prosecutions where there is a dispute between medical experts and no other important evidence. This week a number of parents who lost their living children through having them forcibly adopted, after their removal by the family courts, are appealing to get their children back.

Friday 5th March 04.

Today Eilish's school is closed because it's polling day. Schools certainly don't assume two working parents in their arrangements. I think they should be compelled to provide some sort of fun club day care during all these 'inset' days – a mysterious term which means all kinds of things but no school.

Saturday 6th March 04.

It always seems to be the same. Robert is determined to row with me every

Saturday. He'd been drinking in the afternoon with a friend who has been visiting. I really don't think he can hold his booze. Anyway, Georgina, our baby sitter, pointed out that I'd got the brochure for Sheffield High School for Girls. It was sitting on my desk. He had an immediate loss of temper and tried to rip it up. I told him that I was conducting a comparative analysis of where children end up – it's called 'destinations' in the brochure, and provides a list of where children go: eg. Eilish Hogan, Medicine. London, UCL, and so on. I made it clear that I was going to look at the local State provision too. Robert claims that Tapton's 6th form (a State school) has the best results in Sheffield. I made it clear that I hadn't *decided* anything and that I was merely doing some research to find out what the differences are between schools. For example, I was interested to see that Sheffield High School sends most of its pupils to local Universities: Leeds, Liverpool, Newcastle and Sheffield; however, he wouldn't listen to me and was really horrible. No doubt he'd have been worse if his friend hasn't been here visiting; so much for small mercies. I pointed out his gross hypocrisy in condemning private education when he had been the beneficiary of it himself. Though his particular private school does sound extremely repugnant he probably wouldn't have got his place at Nottingham to study English, at a time when the department there was super trendy, or his first-class degree and prizes without his hot-house start.

Sunday 7th March 04.
Robert is being insufferable. He is bad tempered again. He is shouting because I gave Eilish a drink of milk in leak-proof cup when we'd agreed that we'd have no more drinks upstairs, but she'd pleaded with me and said she'd not had a drink since swimming – which was hours ago. He is a bad tempered bastard. I need for my own sanity and future happiness to leave this relationship. With two children in tow this is a daunting prospect.

***

There was a fairly interesting piece in *The Observer*, which suggested that lack of co-operation and communication between midwives and obstetricians is actually contributing to infant mortality. The piece hinged

around the sad loss of Karen and Wayne Doyle. Karen, admitted to the maternity unit of the Royal Cornwall Hospital, felt that something wasn't right and by the time she had an emergency Caesarean the baby was dead. Belinda Phipps of the National Childbirth Trust discussed the palpable tension in some units between midwifery and medical staff; however, she felt that midwives should have immediate access to a consultant obstetrician as the current system of midwives having to bleep the junior doctor causes unacceptable delays in women being seen by a specialist with experience. The other big problem she identified is simply a shortage of midwives, who have to dash between a number of women in labour.
I shall certainly be having a home-birth. In fact, by the time I've made a cup of tea and run a bath it will all be over if it's as quick as my last one.

Monday 8th March 04.
I had an enjoyable session with my therapist, mainly talking about how difficult I find Robert to be with. When I described several incidents we've had recently – his anxiety about what questions Eilish *might* ask over meals which make him super-tense, the toast incident and others I probably haven't mentioned, he immediately diagnosed him as having 'escalating thought disorder', a form of obsessive compulsive disorder. I found it really confirming to talk to someone who seemed to understand how wearing it is living with Robert's stuff. I'm suffering from anxiety about what Robert will get uptight about next syndrome! Okay, that's not a very good joke! But it occurred to me that perhaps that's why I'm feeling so tired, that it's bound up with my lack of relaxation around Robert….
I also told my therapist about my escape fantasy, the reoccurring one about how I'll leave Robert. But I also told him that I think I'm pregnant. I'm feeling very confident about it this month for no particular reason. He described my situation as 'complex' and it certainly is.

Tuesday 9th March 04.
I'd only been back here a matter of hours when he shouted at me again. Although I agreed to the general principle of no drinks upstairs I think we must be flexible (I'd said this on Sunday) so I let Eilish have a Ribena in a leak proof cup. But the irony of my so doing was that I was trying to keep us to the routine to please him – HIS ROUTINE – THE ROUTINE

HE HAS IMPOSED ON US – and I knew letting her downstairs for a drink would make us late…
So here I am: forty-three years of age, living in a luxurious house but ranting about Ribena! How did I get to this point, I ask myself? What bizarre quirk of fate has led to this? And Robert – how did I end up with someone who cares more passionately about enforcing a trivial house rule than making me happy? Why couldn't he make his point in a gentle way? Why can't he just care about me a lot more? I feel so short-changed… I get no opportunity to relax it feels. Perhaps this really is why I've been feeling so tired lately?
Anyway, this incident gave me my opportunity to suggest, forcefully this time, that he sees a cognitive behavioural therapist – and he's found a number and promises to phone tomorrow.

***

Now I've had a chance to calm down, I still feel that we have enough to justify saving. On Sunday, for example, we had such a nice time at the pool with the children and we swap back and forth. Eilish is courageous now diving through the machine-generated waves and sliding down the flumes. Emile has gained in confidence but still, generally, prefers the baby pool (which has a mini-waterfall, fountain and jacuzzi) with little forays into the big one. I enjoy pottering with the baby or swimming about with Eilish. But then, after a thoroughly pleasant day, he'll blow our harmony over something utterly trivial – me giving Eilish milk, on this occasion. He says she "manipulates me". I retort that I think it's reasonable for a thirsty six-year-old to be given a drink if she asks for one. I love Eilish and I only want to make her happy. I rather think he's doing more "manipulating" than she is… She's too young to be sophisticated at manipulating; she's just expressing basic needs such as thirst.

Friday 12th March 04.
Today my cervix is like a firm, unripe, tropical fruit, slightly irregular in shape with an uneven surface. When I'm ovulating it's like some kind of underwater creature or plant, fleshy, wet and open – waiting for its prey. Certainly, trying to get pregnant has made me much more aware of its rhythm and movement.
Unfortunately, I'm having doubts about my conception. Yet again, I've

had a slight stomach upset. I seem a bit prone to them. So now I'm thinking what I mistook for early signs of pregnancy is not that…

Saturday 13th March 04.
There was one of those very disturbing pieces in the newspaper today. The headline was *'Caesarean refusal' mother in jail* and was accompanied by a mug-shot style photo of the mother in which she looked more than a little deranged. The case is described as 'a test of new state and federal legislation expanding the definition of human life.' Melissa Rowland, age 28, is accused of "depraved indifference to human life" for refusing the C-section – though she denies this. What is significant about her case is that she did not want to keep the twins. The baby girl was given up for adoption and the boy was stillborn. Is she is being punished for her lack of maternal instinct? The absurdity of the case is evident in the language used: 'if she is convicted of causing her *unborn* son's death, Ms Rowland could face life in prison…' How can you kill something that is *unborn* – it's ridiculous? Lynn Paltrow, of Advocates for Pregnant Women, commented: "In the US citizens including pregnant women have the right to refuse unwanted medical treatment, and apparently Utah prosecutors don't believe that applies to pregnant women."
It's like some kind of science-fiction nightmare – the idea that I could be forced into having *life-threatening surgery* against my will. Foetal risks are so difficult to interpret and most women who refuse the offer of a C-section go on to deliver healthy babies naturally. Ultimately, women must be allowed to make decisions, even bad ones, about their own medical care as a basic human right.
On the other hand, I know many women who have regretted having abortions. Therefore, I'd be pleased to see more resources available for women contemplating abortions so that they could be offered supportive counselling: not counselling by Born Again Christians aimed at talking them out of it, but friendly non-judgemental support that would allow women to discuss their despair and help them explore the irrevocable nature of the decision. I feel that many women, feeling alone and in anguish, given this extra support, might find the strength to keep their babies… After all, a lot of abortions are made in the midst of emotional turmoil – a turmoil that does pass.

Please don't misinterpret these remarks: I am pro-choice. Indeed, I think abortion should be available on demand, rather then on a doctor's recommendation (since some doctors are supportive and some not). Nevertheless, it's sad to talk to women who, like my former au-pair, still weep almost daily for the baby they didn't have.

Sunday 14th March 04.
My sister, Lisa, harangued me over the phone when I told her that I'm not using contraception. She said I was being "irresponsible" for trying to get pregnant when my marriage was unstable. "I just want one more little baby", I replied whiningly…

Friday 19th March 04.
The last ever episode of *Sex and the City*, ended with the theme of love. Poor Miranda, who didn't fancy living in Brooklyn anyway, ends up with her husband's mother, a dipsomaniac who has just had a stroke, moving in with them. Her future looks full of obligations and worry and love, of course. Being single looks more attractive as Carrie falls for 'Big', who has finally realised he can't live without her, and Samantha regains her libido after chemotherapy. Meanwhile, Charlotte and husband have a meeting with the expectant 'parents' of the child they are intending to adopt, poor rural folk, who announce that they have changed their minds and want to keep the forthcoming baby. Charlotte's ghastly whiney gay friend asserts that he knows people who can procure a Guatemalan kid for $100 bucks! It's a throw-away line and the morality of rich New Yorkers buying babies from those impoverished is not explored. The episode ends with them finding out that they have been allocated a Chinese baby from an adoption agency – Charlotte weeps for joy. In *Friends,* the theme of adoption continues as Monica and Chandler clean their apartment in readiness for their meeting with the adoption social worker. This is an important meeting as apparently she can keep them off every adoption list in the State, we are told.

Saturday 20th March 04.
The Guardian had three baby related pieces in it. One was a small report about a woman who'd gone binge drinking at a nightclub leaving her baby

alone in her car for five hours, without food or drink or adequate clothing in cold winter weather – I was curious to know if the baby had a blanket but the article didn't say. Then she'd attempted, drunk, to drive but reversed into another car when attempting to leave. District judge, Alan Berg, at Manchester magistrates court described the incident as a 'shameful episode of child cruelty.' Admonishing her he said, "You, in my view, abandoned all your natural instincts and responsibilities… to have a good time." (If she'd done the same thing because she'd had no childcare and had to go out to work I wonder if the judge would have been less harsh? Clearly, that her 'instinct' was to go out and *enjoy herself* was particularly reprehensible…) All the same, I was surprised by the stiff three-month custodial sentence, which won't exactly help her become a better mother…

Another slightly disturbing story, but completely different, had the title *Baby Given Eight New Organs in Record Transplant*. The baby, Alessia, was born with smooth muscle disorder (megacystis microcolon syndrome) preventing normal functioning of her stomach, intestines and kidneys. She'd already been operated on a dozen times in Italy before being flown to Miami, where she underwent the major surgery and two subsequent procedures. Her belly was described as 'criss-crossed by scars…' She was six kilograms when she had the major surgery (13Ibs). The kidneys were each described as 'the size of a walnut, and her intestine the width of spaghetti'. It was not stated if she has *Downs Syndrome*, but looks as though she might have from the photo – certainly, 'the toll exerted from illness and successive surgeries remains unclear', this is rather ambiguous but could mean that she'll reject the organs, the size of the transplant relative to the patient's body weight increases the risk of rejection. It will entail her taking drugs for the rest of her life – or it might mean that she will suffer from permanent ill health. I wonder about the ethics of such experimentation, the suffering of the infant, their quality of life, and about consultants who think they are God.

The last piece in the 'Comment and Analysis' section had Kate Figes, an eloquent whinger about how dreadful motherhood is, talking with Ellie Lee, a lecturer in social policy at the University of Kent and author of a book on abortion. Lee starts off by questioning whether the increasing tendency (in *The Guardian*, at least) to depict motherhood as a miserable

ordeal is either accurate or helpful? Figes, in turn, talks about 'adjustment' and 'many women feeling overwhelmed' und unable to marry their immediate needs with the immediate needs of the child. It's a 'bit of a shock and exhausting', she asserts. All I can say is – it is! it is! Nonetheless, that's not the same as feeling miserable about it.
Lee accuses Figes of 'pathologising motherhood.' Figes retort is quite true of my experience of talking with mothers: that women are often isolated and lacking sufficient support networks, perhaps they don't even know their neighbours; furthermore, new mothers lack confidence in their ability to look after their baby.
I got the impression, reading the exchange that Lee isn't actually a mother, but I could be wrong…

Sunday 21st March 04.
Another week has sped by. I have no time or peace. Eilish has just had her seventh birthday party, though her birthday is on Monday. The party bus was a great success. It had a disco on the top floor, a ball pit, and sand pit on the ground floor and a big slide. The children went absolutely wild and there was lots of high-pitched screaming. All the parents arrived exactly on time to collect them at 4pm. Eilish's uncle has just set up her lap-top (my present to her) with a stunning array of games, one of which includes animals in a jungle who play different instruments allowing musical compositions to be created by clicking on different animal configurations; it's very impressive.
Eilish will open her presents tomorrow after I get home from work. Unfortunately, she says she wants us to eat at Pizza Hut! I was trying to steer her to an Italian child-friendly restaurant, which has a better ambience and a decent wine list…

Monday 22nd March 04.
Eilish had her new best friend round for a play session. I didn't like the girl, which made the meal out a bit of an ordeal. It was fun watching Eilish open her gifts and we had a cake with candles – of course. Emile was brattish at the table, chucking things on the floor and squealing (he was probably over-stimulated by the appalling pop music). I've got some sort of virus or food poisoning or something so perhaps my patience was

impaired as a consequence of feeling off-colour. Eilish says her friend gets a little "giddy" when she's excited. Eilish was well behaved.
I can hardly believe my little baby is a big strong strapping girl. Recently, she's stopped throwing herself into my arms when I get home from work and I have to say I really miss it when it doesn't happen, even though I tend to get an ecstatic greeting from Emile. Eilish and I are having an annual holiday – just the two of us – and I have to say I'm really looking forward to it. I had to fight for it, as Robert didn't like the idea at all. But I really want some special time alone with her, and it means a lot to me that he backed down.

Tuesday 23 March 04.
It's time to have more baby making sex. Although Robert has been calm and loving for a fortnight now, I can't put my hand on my heart and say that I am feeling in love with him again after the recent spate of rows. I wonder if my sister isn't right? I have so little time left if I am still fertile – we haven't got time to 'stop-trying' while we sort things out. We haven't actually even got a time in our diaries when we could both attend a Relate session without children in tow…

Saturday 27th March 04.
It's all over. I was lying back on the bed and Robert was down there between my legs and I found my mind wandering. Well this happens from time to time, you assert- it's normal - of course! But my mind did not wander to Brad Pitt, or to some other fabulous testosterone filled hunk, but to where to plant more Eucalyptus trees in the garden! I can't believe I was thinking about gardening while he was *down there*. What's happening to me? What happened to the eroticism of our relationship?

Sunday 28th March 04.
Soaps – baby Emma did re-enter the story line of *Friends*. Ross was appalled to discover that she'd been entered in a baby beauty pageant, though became less argumentative on discovering she'd won $1,000.

Monday 29th March 04.
Well, tonight I know we won't be having sex after having had conception

sex from Tuesday to Sunday. Today's only day 16 of my cycle but we've decided I'm probably ovulating earlier than we'd previously thought.

Saturday 3rd April 04.
Robert has just handed me a flute of champagne having bought me a dozen red roses this morning. He's booked a table at one of Sheffield's best restaurants for this evening. Occasionally, I think things might work out…

Sunday 4th April 04.
In *Friends* Chandler and Monica have their adoption interview – that is a meeting with the pregnant women who has selected them as the adoptive family. It's a weird prospect summed up my Chandler's quip made when he is imagining the forthcoming encounter, "Hi I'm Chandler, may I have the human growing inside you?" The serial numbers of the case files ensure total anonymity; however, the twist is that the donor has written down the wrong case number. Consequently, at interview when she says she'd delighted to be giving her baby to a minister and a doctor, Chandler (an advertising agent) and Monica (a chef) are rather taken aback. There's a further twist when Monica and Chandler decide not to correct her misconception, but then have second thoughts as the mother deserves to know to who her baby is really going to, they decide. The mother is angry about the deceit and Chandler is forced to grovel that he'll learn to be a good father and describes Monica is "a mother without a baby", a bit of an odd concept which presumably means she has lots of natural instinct.

Monday 5th April 04.
My optimism is short-lived. We're back to the "it's my tone of voice" stuff again. Robert, my beloved, accused me of making a huge mess in the kitchen (actually I think it was our guests) but I merely quipped, in response to the accusation, that having been out of bed for only five minutes I didn't appreciate being criticised. And that was it. Six hours later he was still sulking (I hadn't raised my voice or shouted or snapped). I made numerous attempts to lift his mood throughout the day but he wasn't budging. Eventually at 7.30pm when I attempted to engage him in conversation, he was totally provocative and abrasive and I lost my

temper. I really don't think I can continue to live with this man. If I don't respond in *exactly the right way* the mood is blown and I'm sick of it. But, no man no baby. And no man, lots more unsupported child-care…

Monday 12th April 04.
Having done an Easter egg hunt in the garden yesterday (on my own as Robert didn't want to move from the sofa) I ended up doing another one as a friend arrived with a basket of Easter chicks (toy ones) and eggs (and chocolate beetles), which she hid in the garden. Needless to say, the children were all hyper after the chocolate so we whisked them off to an adventure playground to let off steam.

Tuesday 13th April 04.
This diary is finished. This relationship is finished. I've said this before but now I believe it. I'm living with someone who is constitutionally incapable of being happy.
I typed out a long list of the ways he drives me crazy. It's the cumulative effect which is so oppressive. After reading the list I think I should just get out… I don't think Robert is capable of being the kind of man I'd like to be with.

Wednesday 14th April 04.
I sat in the sunshine today with Emile pottering around playing with his sand-pit and it was delightful. Cuddling Eilish at bedtime and reading her stories was lovely. I wonder if I could enjoy being a single parent with two children? I feel so daunted by that prospect.

Thursday 15th April 04.
This is the day I've been refusing to think about. It's time for our chat with the paediatric surgeon about Emile's orchidopexy, a relatively routine operation, but, with any invasive technique, there could be "injury to other structures", as it was euphemistically put. That means they could cut through a blood vessel or damage a vital organ by accident. There's also the risk of post-operative infection – quite a serious risk in most modern hospitals which become septic environments, full of super-bugs (antibiotic resistant bacteria). Then there's the fairly minimal risk of the

general anaesthetic itself. The consultant we saw seemed very gung-ho about the surgery. Now ultra-sound machines are getting so good that can record foetal smiles in the womb why are they not scanning first rather than going straight in? I asked a lot of questions, he was dismissive about scanning but I wished I had pressed further him on the matter… I was fine with the meeting and asked lots of questions and was calm and rational until he got to outlining the risks and showing us the permission form. Then I burst into tears.

Thursday 22nd April 04.

Many kindergarten children burnt to death, trapped in their bus in Basra, Iraq today. It was the work of Jihad suicide bombers. The war is clearly not over.

Ironically, I was trying to have time out and I read the piece relaxing in the 'tranquillity' area of my local Turkish baths – part of my new trying to be less stressed and tired all the time regime.

I wondered afterwards if the steam room followed by icy plunge pool was a good idea? After all, hot and cold baths used to be regarded as a potential abortifacient.

Saturday 24th April 04.

My friend Sarah and her baby Vandon have just left. We've been sitting in the garden virtually all day with the children pottering about. Vandon and Emile fought over two plastic egg-cups and a toy car. Another little visitor, Chester age three, got stuck up a tree. Eilish injured herself twice, requiring antiseptic on the small wounds. Apart from that, the day was very relaxing… Robert is bathing the very dirty children as I write (which is highly unusual as I usually do the bath) but it sounds as though murder is being committed so I should go.

Sunday 25th April 04.

My health club is full of large posters of a woman looking serene and slightly mystical. It's a head and shoulders shot of her looking slightly skywards. The other poster is of a young man leaping between two rocks. The camera angle is looking up at him as he is caught in mid air. Clearly, having a personal fitness instructor (what the posters are plugging) will have a different effect depending on your sex. Women will be serene and men properly masculine…

Monday 26th April 04.

I forgot to mention that the consultant's reply to my letter arrived today. He argues that whilst ultrasound can show an undescended testis in the abdomen it cannot be relied upon to prove there is no testis present. Proving a negative is hard and the risks in missing the testis outweigh the necessity for surgical investigation, he argued. I still find it amazing that there isn't a non-operative scanning technique which is reliable. My little baby under the surgeon's knife – I can't bear the thought of it. No doubt if I insist on getting a second opinion I'll be characterised as unreasonable!

Wednesday 28th April 04.

Robert announced that he's thinking of trying out a type of martial art called Aikido. I almost choked on my food as he's such a lounge-lizard. I just couldn't imagine a couch-potato like him doing anything remotely energetic apart from mowing our grass. Because I do all of the gardening apart from the grass, I won't take pity on him and do it even though he sweats buckets while he does it and then announces he is shattered for the rest of the day. Now I've been working on my fitness, post-virus, I think I could do it without noticing!

Sunday 2nd May 04.

It's a bank holiday weekend and we should all be happy because it's sunny. But Robert is sulking. He gave Eilish a comprehension test this morning and the result was poor, then he overheard her being stroppy (it was a very momentary 'strop') just before lunch, Emile was also fractious, then she didn't finish her lunch (which always enrages him). Ioana didn't like the buffet; she nibbled on bits and pieces, pulling faces at the strange tastes. Robert hates "fussy eaters" so this couldn't have helped his mood either (he later acknowledged that this "enraged him"). Ioana doesn't like cheese – the lunch was a cheese board and a hot cauliflower cheese (he'd forgotten about her cheese thing) with salad (which she didn't like) and babaganoush (a paté made from aubergines), which she also rejected along with the homous (a paté made from chick peas). She wouldn't eat her potato as it had been adulterated with the cheese sauce from the cauliflower cheese he'd originally served to her because he'd forgotten about her cheese thing. She managed to eat a few cherry tomatoes, bits of cucumber and some bread.

When I was chatting with the health-visitor this week (she'd called to find out how our session in paediatric surgery had gone) I told her about the food war. She thought that making Eilish sit over her lunch for more than half-an-hour would be "counter-productive". So after half-an-hour, to try a compromise, I suggested we go to the park and she could finish the plate on her return. Personally, I don't care if she finishes a plate or not but he insists she should eat everything and if I don't "support him" he'll shout or sulk or both, (why am I with this man I ask myself at such moments? Oh why?). So to avoid him shouting I suggest this compromise.

We had a lovely time in the park (including ice creams and a visit to the ducks…) and I forgot all about Robert's bad mood while I was out with Ioana and the children. On my return home I sat Eilish down at the table in front of her plate; however, at that very moment, I remember it's Izzy's birthday party – but not a normal party – it's a trip in a mini-bus to an adventure playground so we can't be late. They are setting off at three o'clock and it's seven minutes to three. I scream at Eilish to leap into the car, "no, you haven't got time to brush your hair", "no, you haven't got time to change your shoes", I yell…. I drive carefully but swiftly and, luckily there is little traffic, we get there on the dot. They are all waiting outside the house – phew! When I return home, Robert is in a black mood and accuses me of "undermining him". I stayed uncharacteristically calm, and gave a really fulsome apology, "I'm really sorry I totally forgot about the party, but I assumed we'd both like her to go to it, and I know I promised I'd get her to ask her to eat the plate, but because of the mini-bus we couldn't get there late" etc. etc…. I find myself grovelling over something I think is ridiculous in the first place – a tiny scrap of food left on her plate is an irrelevance! But it's not irrelevant to him and now he is doing a super-sulk, which means he won't even talk to me. He will not accept my apology graciously. He now wishes to be "left alone" and I am left fuming and feeling as though I'd like to punch him… One of us is

insane and I genuinely believe it's *him*, not me!
Anyway, I've now calmed down writing this and intend to enjoy the sunshine and the rest of the day…

***

The Observer newspaper has a piece under the heading of 'Caesarean controversy'. Actually, it has two pieces both of which are pro-Caesarean. What is the controversy? NICE (The National Institute for Clinical Excellence) has suggested that the 9,000 or so C-sections performed each year purely at the 'mother's request', rather than for medical reasons, shouldn't be done from the N.H.S. purse. These women should be dissuaded from having the C-section and counselled towards having a natural birth, the report suggests. Perfectly sane and rational you might think? Why would any sane person want to have a major operation when it is clinically unnecessary? However, this is an outrage apparently because the NICE committee report recommendations will impinge on 'consumer choice'. I'm not sure when having unnecessary elective surgery became a matter of 'consumer choice' but clearly I am out of touch.
One of the articles was written by a woman who had a phobia about having a natural birth (perhaps I should use the term 'vaginal delivery' rather than the term 'natural birth' – I'm sure she'd take any drugs on the go). She'd had a traumatising experience when she was young and had never recovered and although perfectly healthy had two very expensive, and completely unnecessary, C-sections. Despite the risks associated with C-sections, 'infection, blood clots and bladder injuries', she remained undaunted. Friends and acquaintances 'had ended up agonised, incontinent and so deeply traumatised by their natural deliveries that they likened them to a car crash' she asserts, as though C-section is a trauma and pain free alternative, which clearly it is not!
This woman did make one sensible point in her article: 'Isn't it ironic that, instead of placing the emphasis on avoiding Caesareans in the cases when women really *don't* want them… the NICE report is targeting the tiny handful of women who do?' I can see that making elective C-sections harder to get will save a lot of money so it's a logical cost cutting exercise. Stopping women who don't want a C-section from being coerced into one would also be a way of saving money – but isn't this cutting into the bread

and butter of obstetrics? You're a few days over your 'due date', the scan shows that the baby is fine, nevertheless your waters are broken and if that doesn't start labour you're given drugs intravenously, no progress? Well it's episiotomy and ventouse or the C-section for you then… And all because the baby wasn't ready to come yet. We are all different and some babies come slightly early and are fine. Others come slightly late and are fine. Policies that dictate automatic intervention after then baby is one week over its 'due date', for example, would have to be revised – perhaps a few obstetricians would be out of a job. I can't imagine so many would be needed after a thorough policy review. Certainly, having critical scrutiny of obstetric regimes would be a challenge for the profession especially if it led to a reduction of services; the current focus is less controversial….

***

The party is now over. Eilish was well behaved and charming I was told. On returning home she was asked to finish off the scraps of lunch she had left. She is now sitting in the kitchen weeping in front of the plate of food she does not want to eat. Robert is shouting at her and *I want to kill him…*

Monday 3rd May 04.
Last night I told Robert that henceforth Eilish would only sit at the table for a maximum of 20 minutes after the rest of us have finished our meal and that when we have a buffet lunch she'll choose her own plate. This caused a row, of course, but I will not relent. I told him that I though the way he'd treated Eilish was abusive.

Tuesday 4th May 04.
Robert and I had our first *Relate* marriage counselling session today. It was uneventful as it was an opportunity, primarily, for the counsellor to familiarise herself with what we regard as our problems. I gave her the list I'd typed – she said it felt "overwhelming" – "that's what it feels like being swamped by all Robert's stuff", I replied. He said the problem was Eilish's behaviour (though when he gave an example of her outrageous behaviour, the counsellor responded that it sounded like "typical behaviour" for the age. At least she has challenged his obnoxious

assertions that she is "abnormal"). I hope this is going to be a *wake-up call* for Robert. He was loving afterwards and held my hand on the way home.

Friday 7th May 04.
I woke up covered in blood. Despite the fact that I've been failing to get pregnant for over a year, I felt upset. If only I could *know for sure* that my fertility was over then I could bury this desire to have another baby and get on with rehabilitating my career and enjoying Eilish and Emile.

Saturday 8th May 04.
I was sitting in my study and knew Robert and Emile had returned from the supermarket because I could hear them all along the street singing the last line of *Wind the Bobbin Up*, over and over, "all day long, all day long"…. Emile just delights in singing now. It's so lovely to have their return announced by the sound of happy singing.

Wednesday 18th May 04.
Emile, now age nearly two and five months, planted his first tree today. He dug the hole and popped it in and then shovelled the compost into the hole and patted it down… I'm not convinced he could conceptualise what he'd done though.

Thursday 19th May 04.
Eilish was leaping up and down on her trampoline. She was slightly overexcited having just had a play session with Izzy who had come to view the garden with her dad, Mike. She fell off; she often does this. But when she stood up, in tears, her lower arm was horribly contorted. I hadn't heard the crack but Izzy's dad said he'd heard it. Mike took over, asking for ice for a compress, and then carrying her to his car. I was far too distraught to drive and Robert doesn't.
Accident and Emergency at the local children's hospital was far nicer than I'd expected, having only sampled the adult version before. There were bunnies and whatnot and she was fixed up with a video of *Snow White* within an hour of arriving. She was given a row of smiley faces – on the left they smiled and on the right they looked more and more miserable and had tear drops. She was asked to point at the one that indicated her level

of pain. I don't know if it was the catheter being inserted, or if it was a mild shock reaction, but I nearly passed out. A nurse had to get me a glass of water and a seat and I was hot and dizzy for a while.

Eilish was asked four or five times how she'd hurt herself. I wasn't sure how to interpret this – either as a sign of general chaos, or as part of a policy to deliberately question children repeatedly in search of discrepancies in their account of the cause of the accident, which might point to child abuse. I suspect it was just chaos.

Eilish was very calm and so was her friend Izzy (and Izzy's dad) but I was blubbering by this point…

As anyone who has been in hospital knows, everything seems rather slow. We had to wait to see a "bone specialist" and then wait to get an X-ray, and then wait to see someone who could explain the X-ray, then wait for a temporary bandage, then wait for a decision about whether or not she'd receive treatment immediately (dependant on the severity of other cases arriving), then wait for a place on the ward (when it became evident she wouldn't receive treatment there and then) and so on. Then on the ward, we had to wait for a sling, without which she was not supposed to use the toilet. Mainly, we were waiting for more pain relief and for all the noise and hustle and bustle to calm down so I could settle her for sleep. There were the inevitable forms to fill in too.

The next day was more of the same except that because she was due to have a general anaesthetic she was not allowed to eat or drink anything so she was progressively more hungry, thirsty and cranky.... Above all, she was bored. They had thought that they might need to operate surgically because of the nature of the two broken bones but ended up just manipulating them back into place, consequently the operation was fairly quick and the worst bit, from my point of view, was waiting for her to come round after the general anaesthetic. I tried to imagine what life would be like without her (not a good plan). Then there was a lot more waiting to find out if she'd be released to come home or not. The nurses said she'd be discharged in an hour then the registrar told me she'd be kept in overnight. I was absolutely shattered by the time we hopped into a taxi. Then after we'd been home for an hour she thought her fingers were swelling and said she was in a lot of pain so Robert whizzed back to the hospital in a taxi with her. Suddenly, I was feeling very grateful not to be a single parent anymore…

Saturday 22nd May 04.
Eilish is remarkably cheerful already and has not asked for any painkillers. In *Music Play Time* her music teacher wrote musical notes on her plaster cast, and I gather she was the centre of attention. Fortunately, she was able to join in with some singing…

Sunday 23rd May 03.
There were two disturbing pieces in today's *Observer* but for completely different reasons. The first was about physically abused pregnant women – fairly rare you'd have thought. Men feel protective towards pregnant women, don't they? However, the Confidential Enquires into Maternal Death (which examines why women and babies die during or after childbirth) estimates that a stunning 12 per cent of women suffer some form of abuse *during their pregnancy*. The Home Office puts the figure at 16 per cent! Apparently, domestic violence can be triggered by pregnancy. I supposed that's not so surprising for the post-natal period in which no one is getting enough sleep – tempers can get frayed; however, this article suggests that simple jealousy is a trigger as women get lots of attention whilst pregnant from family members and health-care professionals. Astrid Osbourne, Consultant Midwife, at the Elizabeth Garrett Anderson and Obstetric Hospital, London, is quoted as saying: 'It is all about power. During the pregnancy the woman is the focus of attention. It is too simplistic to say the man is jealous – it is more to do with him thinking he is losing control over her… he thinks she is no longer his property.' A small qualitative study (by Dr Gillian Aston of King's College, London) found that a third of women had 'suffered violence' at the hands of their partners during the six weeks after giving birth.
The other disturbing article was about *Fathers 4 Justice*, who recently supported one father who had been having difficulty getting access to his six and eight year old daughters (the couple separated when the children were two and four). The mother in this case had made 'unfounded allegations of assault' (the use of the word 'unfounded' is interesting, perhaps she was not sufficiently articulate?) and had not co-operated with access orders. Last week, High Court, Judge Bracewell, of the family

division granted custody of the children to the father. A victory for *Fathers 4 Justice* but a good decision for the children? The younger child would have no recollection of her father. The article said, 'Now, having lived for most of their lives with a mother described as "implacably hostile" to the father, these two small girls will be living with him". How could that be good for either of the children? The baby would not recognise the strange man and the older child would either have recall of the former violence or have been convinced by her mother that he is an absolute bastard. Let's not ask what he did to engender the implacable hostility (something bad, I suspect), let's just ask if this is a good decision for the children? No, no, no. Surely this is punishing a woman who flouted access orders *at the expense of her children*?

Sunday 30th May 04.
Whilst at the children's hospital, I bought a little yellow newborn cardigan for my friend Sarah who's pregnant. She'd been trying for a while (but probably not quite as long as me). Now I wonder whether to wait until after she's had the tests or even until after she's had the baby before I give it to her. Some people are superstitious about receiving baby things before the birth. I'll take advice from a mutual friend.

Monday 31st May 04.
It's the end of a long-weekend and tomorrow I must continue with my gigantic pile of marking. Eilish has had loads of extra attention. Her classmates have showered her with gifts! Having broken bones has some compensations.

Tuesday 1st June 04.
Three of my students, on one particular course I teach on healing practices, have written their essays in infertility and the pros and cons of treatment. I hadn't realised that by some definitions I am now defined as 'infertile': this being a person who has had regular sex for a year without conceiving. *Oh my God, I'm infertile!*

Thursday 3rd June 04.
Twice this week I've worked a ten-hour day, trying to get all my marking

done. Yesterday I got a call from Eilish's holiday club telling me to come and get her as she was discovered to have nits. Then of course I had to spend over an hour combing them out, and then again this morning for an hour, to make sure she was clear. That's on top of all this bloody work... At least Ioana, our new au-pair, has settled in well and seems very content playing with Emile when he's not at the nursery. It will be very strange next week going from being frantic, (the deadline for marks is Monday), to being on holiday with Eilish (we are going to *Center Parcs* – just the two of us – for our annual bonding session); however, this week she's seeing her grandparents. She's just been collected by my ex mother-in-law's housekeeper, and whisked off to London. I know London Zoo is on tomorrow's agenda...

Sunday 6th June 04.

This Sunday's *Observer Review* had a big article all about how it's okay to give up work and become a full-time mother. It was a feel-good piece essentially. One of the women who had crossed-over said she had 'no desire to spend time with "shallow people who get all their self-esteem from work" (ouch!). The article takes a swipe at New Labour for harassing women into employment. How about some measures to enable women, who want to, to stay at home, requests the piece. The article also highlighted the endemic discrimination in the workplace, claiming that whilst 63% per cent of medical students are women, 60% of law students and 55% per cent of business students are women, only 20% of medical consultants are women, 37% of solicitors are women and 32 of the FT top 100 companies have no women on their boards... 'We used to blame these kinds of figures on the glass ceiling. But the talk today is all about the 'maternal wall' ... you are generally blocked from doing the kind of job that is generally defined as high-powered', the article asserts. Nevertheless, even though many women are managing to hang on to their high-powered job after motherhood, the article claims that many others are choosing to leave for enhanced quality of life. Juggling a demanding job with motherhood is a generally miserable business, it is suggested. (There was no discussion of paternal responsibility in all this).

The decision, to opt out of employment, is the preserve of the privileged. These educated women have partners who can keep the family with one income – not my situation, unfortunately; otherwise I'd be out of the workplace like a shot! That's not a glib remark; it's true.

I've been trying to negotiate a part-time contact for months now but my manager is as slippery as soap. Just when I thought we'd got an agreement about my teaching load, she volunteered me for something at a public meeting, which we had never discussed. Now she's out of the country overseeing an academic franchise so I can't discuss it with her... I am feeling very angry.

Anyway, I'd quite like to make it to Professor before I quit, which will be harder on a part-time contact, of course. I appreciate that I am expressing contradictory feelings about this subject. After a gruelling week during which I have barely had time to see the children opting out does seem preferable!

Friday 11th June 04.

I've just returned from a mid-week break in Sherwood Forest (*Center Parcs*). I have to say I really enjoyed it, if only because of little Eilish's delight at finding our 'villa' next to a small river, which was inhabited by an abundance of squirrels, ducks with ducklings, swans with cygnets and rabbits. One swan in particular was very audacious, knocking on our patio doors with her beak to demand food. Several of the above visited us at mealtimes and Eilish was in ecstasy feeding all the animals... This and the artificial 'beach' at the lakeside were quite enough to keep her happy. We did sample the 'subtropical swimming paradise', which I found, much like lots of municipal, family-orientated, swimming baths around the country, to be rather noisy, crowded, and not 100% clean. It had the ubiquitous flumes (which Eilish wasn't allowed to use because of her broken arm) and a 'rapids' ride which would have been far too scary for her... They are rather overstating its appeal calling it a 'paradise'. While Eilish went to a couple of 'fun clubs' (they lived up to their name), I did have a couple of sessions in the 'Aqua Sauna', which was a slightly kitsch version of a spa. Why kitsch? Well, apart from the naff statues, coloured flashing lights and mock Roman features, all the steam rooms had the same muzak. There was an Indian blossom steam room and a Japanese salt steam room, a Turkish hummum, and so forth, but the 'new age' sound tracks detracted from the themed interiors. (I could put up with music if, for example, the

Japanese steam room was playing Japanese music and so forth). The spa did have a delightful salt-water swimming pool and a restful 'Zen garden'. Anyway, it was relaxing. The most notable thing about the holiday was how many babies there were (except in the spa). There were hundreds of them. I felt so broody… I kept finding myself peeking at them. How I'd love another baby, though juggling the three would be a challenge. It's day ten of my menstrual cycle on Sunday and fortunately I don't need to stay away on Monday night this week so we should be able to get a good run of 'bonking' done again so long as Robert's stamina holds!

Sunday 13th June 04.

The Observer has a follow-up article on stay at home 'power mums'. Today's piece, citing a dubious survey in *Top Santé* magazine, suggests that two out of three women "want to quit work because they are failing to successfully manage the competing demands of work and home… Trying hard – but failing – to achieve a balanced life is the greatest obstacle to women's happiness", asserted the piece. That's certainly my own problem, I feel.

The article did point out that having a choice to agonise over was the domain of the privileged. But do successful career women who opt out necessarily become 'power mums', I wondered? One woman quoted says, "I'm surrounded by them [power mums], treating their children as a management project… thanks to their rich husbands…" (I can't imagine, when I start working part-time, that I'll turn into a 'power mum' – but I might have time to ensure that Eilish's nits are combed out and that she does her homework sheets). On the other hand, 'perhaps some working mothers enjoy the perennial time management and concomitant martyrdom, the sense of purpose, more than they want to let on', suggests Kathryn Flett. Oh, the pain, the pain of it all… No, I don't think we are a bunch of masochists. I imagine really happy working mothers are very good at compartmentalising – better than I am, in fact... If I could just sit at this computer until 7.15 (when Robert will serve food) and enjoy it and not think about the fact I promised Robert I'd introduce Ioana, our new (ish) au-pair, to a more stimulating range of activities for the toddler (Emile) such as leggo, plastercine or painting (they spend a lot of their time together watching videos). Will he suffer arrested development as a result of such neglect? Alternatively, I should not spare a thought for Eilish's nit combing or her reading practice, or her music practice. There is always a list of things to do for the working mother longer than she can actually accomplish. She is always failing, failing, failing.

This article bangs on about 'esteem' gained from work. What about the esteem to be gained from children with nit free hair or a child who knows the words to the song in the school performance? This is very real, and actually it feels more meaningful than having got my marks submitted to the office in time. Okay, I'm a University Reader, and that gives a modicum of status to my tired and flagging ego (though a lot of Universities are run by managers these days who don't care about intellect or research which does not bring with it lots of dosh) but what really pleases me (apart from good book reviews) is seeing that my children's needs are being met and feeling great that I managed to meet them. Oh dear, am I getting preachy? No I'm not self-righteous - quite the opposite, like the majority of working mums, I suspect.

Anyway, neither description of women's need to work in the article or decision not to is very flattering. Women, unlike men, seem to be criticised whatever decisions they make:

If women work – we are too selfish, too egotistical, the child will suffer deprivation and have arrested emotional development, and miss out from lack of 'school gate' social networks.

If women give-up paid work to become full-time mums - we are causing a waste of a good education, and letting the feminist cause down. Why should employers take the notion of equal opportunity seriously when we quit just as we become indispensable to our employer or after a company has invested in our training? Or, alternatively, we will become monster 'power mums' driving our children into early nervous breakdowns with our towering expectations.

If women never develop a career in the first place – we won't be able to sufficiently stimulate the children; we won't have enough self-confidence to kindle self-confidence in our children; we will reproduce patriarchal values which will spoil our daughters' chances to break out of a breeding role.

If women decide to work part-time – we will botch motherhood anyway as we won't be able to keep up with all the minutia of arranging

sleepovers, play sessions, remembering music rehearsals etc. etc., whilst probably working in a fairly menial position, as most part-time workers do not get equal treatment with those who work full-time for the promotions, nicer offices, better equipment, more interesting remits, further training, conference funding, or whatever. And we'll work more than part-time. The cliché is that we'll get the worst of both worlds.
And this is the broadsheet press I'm discussing here.

Tuesday 22nd June 04.
Robert and I went to our Relate session (he flounced out of the last one and refused to see the same counsellor again so I'm not terribly optimistic about the process). This time we've got a man, which may make a difference.

Wednesday 23rd June 04.
I'm having concerns about my seven-year-old's education. The school is actually quite rough. A boy tried to trip Eilish up at the top of a staircase yesterday (making her fall and causing bruising on her back, though it could have been fatal) and then the same boy kicked her in the crotch in the playground later in the day. Then he sauntered off to play with his friends only to return a few minutes later to administer another kick! Such assaults are so common she didn't even tell me. I noticed a boot mark on the crotch of her trousers and questioned her about it and the whole story came out!
There have been several occasions recently when, having been hit by another child, she has reported the incident, but the perpetrators have never been found. Also she has been wrongly accused of all kinds of minor things by children who are plausible liars. Invariably, the truth does not out. I have been left feeling that the school is rather complaisant about such matters. It's hard for a seven year old to be assertive about what really happened.
When I phoned the head-teacher (the first time I've ever phoned her) she got stoppy over my use of the word 'assaulted'. When I mentioned the boot mark on Eilish's crotch as indicating a serious kick she quibbled with me saying that if it was wet and muddy perhaps an imprint could be made quite easily! I was flabbergasted. "Two kicks to the crotch are a bloody

assault you moron," I felt like screaming.
Anyway, today Eilish was accused of "trying to strangle another girl" and it turns out there was some pushing and shoving and that Eilish shoved another girl in an unacceptable manner (the strangulation bit was a lie – this is a girl who constantly lies); however, the timing was very unfortunate as it's the first time she's been accused of anything serious just after I've insisted that I want the boy who assaulted her to be caught. The head teacher even made snide, smug, remarks to my partner about how she was no better than the boy. This was somewhat irksome.
As for Eilish's academic work, her best friends are those who joke about and don't concentrate.... I wasn't very academic myself at her age, so although I'm very worried, I'm more concerned by her attitude. At least I was prepared to try hard, whereas copying her friends, she pretends to be blasé and bored.
I got the biggest shock yet on Tuesday when I attended the children's concert. First, the Ashdell Preparatory School for Girls, all immaculate, gave a magnificent performance – orchestral and also in choir singing (four part harmony). They were very sophisticated and disciplined. Later came the 'pop-choir' from the junior school Eilish is to attend next year, and they looked like a bunch of delinquents and sang badly compared to the Ashdell girls. I'm feeling negative about State education right now... Oh God, I'm turning into one of these middle-class mums always fretting about their children's schooling. I swear I never do it at dinner parties! Am I sacrificing my daughter on the alter of ideology? Unlike Tony Blair, I have a partner who will never forgive me if I send her to a fee paying school.

Thursday 24th June 04.
As well as countless shrubs, I've planted sixteen trees since I we moved into this house, mainly Eucalyptus gunnii and fastigiata (for screening), and fruit trees (the three year old apple trees I planted will actually give a crop this year), which shows a commitment of sorts. I like to think that I'll be enjoying the results of all my planting in ten year's time.

Friday 25th June 04.
Mary, my high-powered ex-mother-in-law, conveyed her disapproval of

my decision to work part-time in an e-mail. She says I'll get 'the worst of both worlds'; it's not like her to use a cliché – I'll have to press her on what she means… She packed off her boys to residential public schools, a fate from which neither ever fully recovered. Another friend of mine, an academic, said the same thing. She says I'll end up working almost full-time anyway but without getting paid for it. I fear she is right.

Saturday 26th June 04.
We have decided to try the *Clearblue Ovulation Test*, which works by detecting a surge in the level of luteinising hormone in urine, which occurs, apparently, between 24-36 hours before ovulation. Conception is most likely to occur in the 48 hours following this detected surge. This is better than being uncertain about my ovulation time we've both decided.

Sunday 27th June 04.
Today's fertility reading was called *'Baby Chase'* and was positive about the benefits of post genetic diagnosis (PGD) for horrible genetic diseases such as sickle cell anaemia or muscular dystrophy. This is for 'pre-implantation' fertilised eggs for those undergoing fertility treatment. This works as part of the normal IVF procedures with embryos of six to eight cells being examined for disease-carrying genes. The Human Fertility and Embryology Authority (HFEA) decide what diseases can be screened for. Peter Braude, Professor of the Centre for Pre-implantation Genetic Diagnosis at Guy's and St Thomas' Hospitals, points out that the options for genetic screening are becoming more sophisticated: "We can already test for serious diseases that strike after 40 years of healthy life, such as Huntington's disease. What if we find the gene that causes a predisposition to Alzheimer's or asthma?" Sounds sensible to implant the fertilised egg that doesn't have the ill-health carrying gene to me – why not? Why is this a moral dilemma? The would-be parents can decide whether to implant or not.
PGS (Pre-implantation genetic screening) can also check for chromosomal abnormalities but this is not normally on offer to women under thirty-five. PGS strikes me as unproblematic. Dr Simon Fishel, director of *Care* in Nottingham (Britain's current largest IVF provider) put the case for it succinctly: 'When you produce an egg naturally or through

IVF, you get a random number of eggs that are abnormal… If I have 10 of your embryos I am allowed in the UK to put two of them back [during IVF] – but there is a good chance that I may not pick the two good ones." Think of the poor couples that might have managed a successful pregnancy if this screening were in place as a norm. The current system of not screening seems irrational, given the emotional and physical pain and financial costs involved.

Monday 28th June 04.
Robert went into town to buy the ovulation test and a tourist guide to The Netherlands, but he only took 30.00 pounds with him, and as the ovulation test was a surprising £20.00 he returned home only with the travel guide.

Tuesday 6th July 04.
I've just returned from a long weekend in Amsterdam with Eilish, my seven-year-old daughter. She listed the "pussy-cats in the street", roads that turn into bridges, the play areas in the Vondelpark and house-boats as her favourite things about the city.
Graham, our host, has a little garden flat in the city with a grand piano he let Elish plink-plonk on. He's gay but not so camp he has to live in Amsterdam. Graham is terrific with both children but does not regret his decision not to have one – no, not even slightly, he is very clear on this point.
Having, on my last visit, spent all my time in museums, I decided to do all those other things… Graham took Eilish shopping while I popped into the *Seksmuseum,* as Robert, on a previous visit, had been impressed with 'King Dong', who really does have a penis that hangs down to his knees! We also had a canal boat ride and visit to NEMO: the child-friendly science museum. Graham seemed to enjoy all the interactive exhibits as much as Eilish. We visited another city (Deventer) for contrast, saw an arts festival (comprising mainly huge dinosaurs and aliens, created by stilt-walkers which terrified Eilish). We went to a market, shopped at de Bijenkorf (their equivalent of Jenners in Edinburgh or Liberty in London, sort of, no actually more John Lewis than Liberty) and attended a garden party (come to think of it, it's not surprising I'm shattered!).
The highlight for me was our three-hour bike tour of the canal belt, with

Eilish sitting on the back of my bike. The tour actually included a bit of the Red Light District too, prompting Eilish to ask, "Why are those ladies wearing bikinis?" I'd told her teacher that the trip would be "educational", but not quite *this* educational…

As Eilish is already acquainted with 'the facts of life', as sex education was quaintly called when I was her age, teaching her the meaning of the word 'prostitute' wasn't too difficult. Her response to my elucidation was a rather poignant "So long as I never have to be one". She glazed over when I started trying to explain about human trafficking and how girls can get trapped and tricked into becoming virtual slaves. Her other new word was 'dildo' (we passed several shop windows full of multi-coloured ones). I didn't go into detail about their use; I think she thinks they are mantle-piece ornaments! I did explain that when her school teacher asked about her trip to Amsterdam it might be interesting if she told the class about how most people cycle everywhere on bicycles, and how a lot of people live on house boats, originally because of a post-war housing shortage, or how Amsterdam, like Sheffield, has got trams.

Incidentally, when I dropped her off at school mid-morning on Tuesday, I did hear her teacher ask her about her holiday, the classroom almost silent with most children straining to hear her reply, "I saw Siamese twins", and indeed she had, at NEMO, the science museum: a peculiar little corner full of ancient bottles of formaldehyde containing various monstrosities.

Thursday 8th July 04.

Robert has been very loving and sensual since my return. This is turning into a very nice week.

Friday 9th July 04.

I used my *Clearblue Ovulation Test* this morning, but there was no surge in the level of luteinising hormone in my urine so I guess I'm not fertile yet this month. This is interesting for me because my sexual peak doesn't seem to be corresponding with my ovulation as I had previously thought – I'm peaking now sexually…

Sunday 11th July 04.

My *Clearblue Ovulation Test* showed a definite surge showing that I'm coming up to my ovulation (in the next 48 hours). So, I'm ovulating later than I thought in my cycle. Indeed, recently we have often missed day 15 and frequently missed 16 and 17. It looks as though we have stopped having sex *just before my ovulation* many months! I wish we'd heard of this test before… Now I feel excited to know that I haven't conceived because we have been missing my ovulation rather than because there is a problem. Suddenly, I feel nervous excitement that I could become pregnant again at any moment.

Thursday 15th July 04.
Now it's just the usual waiting game. Fortunately, we are off for our annual honeymoon. Or 'honeymoon', perhaps I should say, given that it's not my fertile period and I know Robert will be far more interested in the impressive buffets than in languorous love-making sessions. And in any case this is something that having another child might end. Robert's mum and dad have the children for a week every year (with au-pair support, of course). We are off to the island of Djerba in the Mediterranean Sea.

Saturday 17th July 04.
Today's review of Gerhardt's *Why Love Matters: How Affection Shapes a Baby's Brain* may not have done the book justice. It mentions heartrending research carried out on the brains of Romanian Orphans who suffered from profound neglect, left to cry in their cots from birth and denied the opportunity to form 'close' relationships. The researchers found 'a "virtual black hole" where the orbito-frontal cortex should have been', (this is the part of the brain thought to help 'enable' people to 'manage' their emotions, we are told). Then the review leaps from this most extreme deprivation to making ominous pronouncements about using a childminder or a nursery – which might be a 'more momentous decision' than we thought, though precisely why is not spelt out.
There is a hormone, continues the review, called cortisol which is produced in a babies brain when it is distressed, but though levels of cortisol may be 'set' by six months of age no plausible argument is put forward for how this might be predictive of future personality traits – indeed, it is highly reductive to suggest that this hormone has any significant effect. No links are made between every day childcare

provision and the poor Romanian orphans.

The article ends with the highly conservative suggestion that 'The government's unbridled enthusiasm for nursery care means that the most vulnerable children in society end up with the biggest deficit in terms of the quality of their early interactions – precisely the same children most likely to end up with behavioural, educational and social problems later on.' This statement is making a number of misguided assumptions: one is that the infant will be less stimulated by a nursery situation than by their mother at home, and there is no evidence for this. On the contrary, much nursery provision is excellent and staff members quickly become familiar, comforting figures (knocking out the overproduction of cortisol, presumably). The most 'vulnerable' children, presumably those raised in poverty, are precisely those who can't afford to use nursery provision anyway (at the time of writing there is no free nursery provision available for the under twos in England). Therefore, the argument is simply not plausible on any level.

Tuesday 20th July 04.

I'm writing from Jerba, a little island famous for its dates and little else (actually also for the harvesting of sea sponges), off the coast of Tunisia. I'm looking out at a beach of white sand blending into turquoise sea. The burgeoning date palms break the horizon. Being here makes me realise how insanely packed my average week is – no wonder I'm often stressed and exhausted. Here I'm sleeping well and feeling totally relaxed. It's our annual 'honeymoon' holiday… Robert just walked over to me (his lounger is in the sun and mine under the shade of a palm) and I looked up lovingly, and with a smile said, "So you are paying me a romantic visit." "Get real," he replied, grabbing the water bottle (he doesn't make it easy for me to love him).

On a more serious note, I keep seeing him looking lovingly at little babies and toddlers and my heart leaps to my throat. I know he is missing Emile but it's the baby we want, but seem unable to conceive, he's thinking about.

Saturday 31st July 04.

Robert and I went to see *The Story of the Weeping Camel* last night. Not an obvious choice for a Saturday night you might think, as it centred on a rejected camel colt, set in an isolated Mongolian community in the Gobi desert. It was a lovely film and Robert was heartbroken for the poor baby camel, sighing, tutting and moaning every time it cried. And there were a lot of shots of this little camel, abandoned by its mother, plaintively crying out for her. Clearly, he is feeling very broody!

Sunday 1st August 04.
I'm trying to decide whether to read the latest this is what it's like to have a baby book, or not. *Making Babies: Stumbling Into Motherhood,* we are told in the review, views motherhood as 'a place where established identities are being ripped apart, bodies violently altered and relationships put under a potentially fatal strain'. Sounds like compulsive reading to me!

Thursday 5th August 04.
I am one of the 'we can have it all' generation and I have spent much of the last eight years exhausted. By some people's definition, I do have it all. It's all a question of perspective. I have relative success, a big house, two beautiful healthy children, reasonable financial security, an often loving and actively supportive partner (one who loads the dish-washer and does the cooking) but never enough time: to be with my children, to 'clear my desk' (either the one at work or the other at home), to get the laundry done. I feel under constant pressure… and I often crave solitude: just a few moments of peace. And sex? Robert lost his erection last night when Emile started calling out, over and over, from his cot, "I need Robert" and singing *Old MacDonald had a Farm*. The latter is actually very funny as Old MacDonald has "a helicopter", "a crying", and various other accoutrements not in the original version of the song…
Perhaps I come across as fickle? I believe in the principle of State education but have been unable to find a local school I have confidence in (like many parents who have aspirations for their children, no doubt). I'm a romantic who believes in love and commitment and fidelity but who is routinely driven to distraction by the man she lives with. I am daily torn between my real desire to be with my children and a natural inclination to be on my own. I hold incompatible aspirations for myself. And of course, I want this third

child. The more delightful Emile is, the more I want another one.

Friday 6th August 04.
I've had two visitors to the house recently, one is a childless lesbian, who is wonderful with the children, who now wishes she had had a child (some of her friends collaborated successfully with gay men, though some alienated their long-term partners in the process) and, the other, a woman, celibate, who used artificial insemination (through a fertility clinic) to have a baby on her own. She has remained a single parent by choice, but she seems very, very tired. (She's an academic too). I think both of them look at what I have rather wistfully, or what they think I have, which is rather different, so I can't talk about how hard I find living with Robert. He cooks them lovely curries when they come to stay and both tell me how lucky I am to have a man who cooks so well - so how can I explain to them how oppressed I often feel by him?

Saturday 7th August 04.
Emile, who is now two-and-half, cherubic with uncut curly hair, came to me and said "daddy slapped me". He repeated it several times. Clearly, Robert has broken his promise not to use corporal punishment. I feel so angry I could murder him (this impulse is paradoxical).

Thursday 12th August 04.
I decided to read Anne Enright's *Making Babies: Stumbling Into Motherhood.* She describes her pregnancy in a way I didn't really recognise; though I enjoyed her funny take on it. Her description did remind me of some people's irrational reactions. One friend of mine, actually quite a close friend with infertility problems, had just been turned down by an adoption agency at the time of my accidental first conception. She couldn't bring herself to speak to me again after I told her my news. She vanished overnight from my life. It's certainly true that ones pregnancy evokes emotions in others. My ex-husband said he felt "violated" by my decision to go ahead with the pregnancy against his wishes. (He hadn't wanted children, to put it mildly).

Enright says it changed the way she saw people. She started noticing the vulnerable, frail and infirm because of her own feelings of precariousness. I, on the other hand, was blithely indifferent to the seething mass of humanity and continued, fairly much as usual, in my little bohemian cocoon consisting mainly of artists and poets – lots of poets. Before motherhood I was somehow socially inviolate; *no one* would ever attempt to make conversation with me on a bus, for example, except for the drunken lunatic on the top floor who was addressing everybody, and nobody in particular. Afterwards, my I-don't-do-small-talk bubble burst and elderly Scottish ladies, wearing tweed skirts and raincoats, suddenly and audaciously, very audaciously I felt, started engaging me in conversations about the weather or the baby, often beginning with "He's a bonny wee bairn", because she was wearing blue cast-offs. I was thrust into the role of reluctant anthropologist in a world to which I had not formally been privy – that of 'mainstream' Scottish society. (I don't think my previous employment in several university departments counts as being part of 'mainstream' society – universities used to be refuges for clever eccentrics). Motherhood plunges you, although the pregnancy is a rehearsal, into an array of unsought for relationships with the outside world though perhaps, unlike me, you were ready for them?

Saturday 14th August 04.

There was another of those 'I didn't have children because mothers are grotesque' articles in the newspaper today. It's not paranoid to note that the broadsheet press is down on motherhood at present and publishes anyone willing to stand up and say how dreadful it is – even if they haven't actually been through it. Anyone can pontificate about mothers, except women who like being one, it seems. I am not with the *zeitgeist,* unfortunately. We fail to cut the umbilical cord and, shame of shame, we may feel our children 'owe' us something… Damn right, my children owe their very existence to my stubborn decision to continue with both pregnancies, neither of which occurred in ideal circumstances – one in the wake of a crumbling marriage, when I'd just started a new job so I got no paid maternity leave, and the second with a man, who should have been, a short-term fling: now my difficult current partner. Only someone who is not a mother could write this stuff, otherwise she would know that having a close relationship with ones children is the most meaningful part of many women's lives. Men come and go but usually we have enduring relationships with our offspring. I intend to love and sustain my children for as long as they need it. I will be there, I hope, to help care for my grandchildren. We will have lasting, and mutually satisfying, love and friendship. Why not? And why should it end, except by death? Rebecca de Saintonge regards a mother's love as 'quietly, insidiously destructive – controlling, manipulative, demanding' and if any of this is true, how, I'd like to ask de Saintonge, does that differ from any other kind of love? My 'husband' is manipulative, controlling and demanding, in abundance, but not of the children – of me… And parents actually have an obligation to be some of these things, since we are bound to socialise our children (or have them removed by social workers). Mothers are 'insidiously destructive'? That's such an odious generalisation to make. I don't regard childless women as selfish, but one or two, like de Saintonge, have very twisted views of motherhood.

Tuesday 17th August 04.
I'm really enjoying Anne Enright's book, *Making Babies: Stumbling Into Motherhood.* I notice, on the little subject box at the back of the book, that it describes itself as a parenting memoir. This does seem to have become a new genre. Enright's description of her disorientation following the birth is brilliant. When she tries to phone home from the hospital she simply can't remember her own phone number. I couldn't spell my own name, I recall, at one point; that's probably when I wept…

Wednesday 18th August 04.
My socially inept Romanian au pair is bothering me. This morning when I sat at the breakfast table, having had mine earlier, it was just to be with my toddler, Emile. I wanted to hear him speak and watch him eat his breakfast. I wanted to help him; indeed, I wanted to mother him. After all, I am on holiday; I have time to be with my children. I offer him the wrong cereal. Ioana intervenes authoritatively, "No, this is his favourite" she says holding up a box as though English is not *my* first language, though we have only been staying at my father's house for two days and all the cereals are different from the usual ones we have at home. I don't cavil, I defer. Even the cereal itself is a compromise; I actually like him to have fresh fruit for breakfast, but a succession of au pairs have put paid to that and now he demands the dry stuff. She stands over him fussing and

ministering. I say, "Sit down and relax. Eat your own breakfast; I'll do it." But within minutes she is hovering again and looking tense. I am a tense person, but compared with Ioana I am positively supine. She can't see that I am happy simply to be with him. Twice more I suggest that she sit or relax. I don't think she likes me interfering. Too much interfering could make her redundant, I suppose. I try to empathise: she's in a strange house, only here to care for the children. She's probably missing the friends she's made in Sheffield. After breakfast, she whisks him away, without asking me if it's okay, and I am left sitting alone at the breakfast table looking out at the sea.

Thursday 19th August 04.

My step-sister, Gillian, told me that she admires my decision to try to have another child and it made me realise that *no one* had said that before. Surely, I've a surfeit of motherhood with two? Here we are at a family gathering, with her son, Ryan, getting on really well with Eilish: they are splashing around in dad's pool, riding lilos, (Gillian and I are taking turns at life-guard duty). And her daughter, Rachael, just one day older than Emile, lets him kiss her as little boys are told to do. Robert's been supportive, and even uncle-like, with all four children climbing all over him at one point, though he has a rather startled expression in the photo. I *can* imagine myself in a larger family, "But it's not happening" I reply to Gillian, "It's just not happening…"

Friday 20th August 04.

I've been feeling a little churned up. Visiting my father made me think about my mother and thinking about my mother always makes me want to weep. She had a raw deal. She was in pain for a long time before she received a correct diagnosis, and by then it was too late – far, far, too late. She didn't get to see my children. Indeed, she died long ago now. My father was cruel to her. Yes, I think that has to be said. She did not receive the love she should have had. I miss my mum. I wonder if I will ever stop missing her? Mummy, I love you.

Later, Eilish asks me what *Fee Fee* was like, and I take her into my arms and hold her gently, so gently, rocking back and forth, and I stroke her tenderly, and answer, "Like this, she was just like this"…

Saturday 21st August 04.
It's a blood thing. Having babies brings out our animalistic emotions. Robert is infinitely less patient with Eilish than with Emile. Is it just biology?
Perhaps, I'll just have to keep living with this terrible disparity of treatment he meets out to them: not even acknowledging Eilish when she enters a room but being so attentive to Emile – so loving, so demonstrative… When he's unkind to my daughter, I really hate him. I wanted to be able to say 'our' daughter but he virtually ignores her, except to tell her off or to complain about her. It's not his sperm, is it? It's not his blood. Why should blood still matter at the beginning of the twenty-first century, I ask myself? I thought biological determinism has burnt itself out, after a last gasp at the turn of the twentieth century with all that worry about the state of the troops for the Boer War.
I keep telling myself it's because he prefers babies. But if he prefers babies he could be as authoritarian and insufferable with Emile, as he is with Eilish, soon; if that happens I'll have to leave him, because I won't be able to stand it… He's shown signs: shouting at Emile, hurting him by squeezing his little wrists, and shaking him on a couple of occasions whilst shouting ferociously into his face. Emile looks like one of those cherubs in Victorian Classical paintings at the moment with his long curls and chubby perfect body – he just needs the little wings. How could Robert hurt him?
Of course I reacted – what mother wouldn't? When I saw Robert do this, I tried reason: I said shaking could give him brain damage. I tried threatening: I said that it was irresponsible to shake him and that I would tell the health visitor - but what does he do when I'm not around to see? I took Emile into my arms and gave Robert the accusatory look: the look that says if you hurt this baby *I will leave you. I will make you pay for this. I will make you regret it.* The most important communication between husband and wife is often silent. I hope he got the message!

***

When I am feeling positive and optimistic, I tell myself that he'll relax more and stop bullying us all, because even his beloved Emile gets it now when he's wilful. (Poor Emile only threw a cracker on the floor earlier today and Robert was screaming at him). But even when I'm feeling optimistic there is part of me which thinks this is all going to end badly, part of me knows that I will not be able to endure his ultra authoritarian parenting style, part of me that knows that I'm going to end up a single parent again – but this time with two kids in tow and an angry ex hovering in the background.

Monday 22nd August 04.
Do you believe in psychic communication? Sometimes I think Robert wants Eilish dead. There, I've said it. I've brought it out into the open – this insidious hatred that seems to be growing inside him.
Sometimes I *know* he wants her dead. Sometimes, I think he'd just like Eilish gone so we could get on with the important task of enjoying our baby together. Eilish is a lovely child only seven years of age. I don't understand why he can't open his heart to her. I don't understand why he wants her dead.
At this precise moment Eilish is at a 'club'. She's out of the way. Emile's latest nickname is 'Berituse' – don't ask me why: "I'm getting Berituse" he beams, before trotting off to the nursery round the corner. We are a happy couple; we are about to appreciate our son together in the evening sunshine.

Thursday 26th August 04.
Robert's best friend has just become a father. The labour was induced (always a mistake if not for dire medical reasons, I think) after she was just one week overdue. There followed a 40-hour ordeal, culminating with an epidural, episiotomy and forceps delivery. The baby, born at 2am on Tuesday, was very bruised by the forceps and barely breathing. They did not get to hold her as she was rushed away to intensive care where she remains. Patrick told Robert that he'd have wept if he'd spoken to him yesterday, so traumatising was it. They have yet to hold little Esmie who is still in an incubator with a collapsed lung…

Sunday 29th August 04.
I gave my baby sling to my friend Sarah today. She has been visiting with her partner, John, and son, Vandon, who is two, and complained that she hasn't managed to find a comfortable sling (she's twenty four weeks

pregnant now and needs a new sling as Vandon is still in a buggy). I told her how terrific mine was and then it occurred to me to offer it to her – after all, "I'll not need it for at least nine months", I quipped as I handed it over. But I suspect I'll not be using it again now. Somehow it felt like a symbolic act, giving away my beloved baby carrier. All my cupboards and under bed spaces are groaning with baby things I've been unable to give away: baby-grows, vests, little shoes – you get the picture. Soon, I think I'll clear the whole lot out.

***

Little Esmie remains in her incubator in a stable condition. Patrick and Vicki have been allowed to touch her by putting their fingers in a little hole in the side of the box…

Monday 30th August 04.
Little Esmie is "up and down", says Robert. I ask what up and down means and he says he doesn't know…

Wednesday 1st September 04.
Esmie is going home today. Babies are robust little creatures. I've got a little mark above my left eyebrow; it's been there for over four months since Emile biffed me with the sharp edge of a toy. If Emile scratches himself, the wound has completely vanished in a week. It's like magic - baby skin. I am only forty-three but I just don't seem to heal anymore.

Saturday 4th August 04.
My au-pair's Polish boyfriend said I looked "very sexy" and that I didn't look as old as forty. He told Ioana this, not me. I guess that's what we old birds like to hear every now and then.

Sunday 5th August 04.
Robert went to visit Esmie today, and he held her in his arms and stoked her and kissed her little face repeatedly – such an intimate gesture. He says he was in ecstasy. Robert's friends were surprised how she stopped crying as soon as he took her in his arms; he has "the touch".

Monday 6th September 04.
Even though I might be fertile Robert and I were too fatigued to have sex together. At least it was a mutual decision.

Tuesday 7th September 04.
We had our last baby making sex of the cycle today (day 17). This is the time of each month when I imagine having the third; I visualise a tiny newborn baby in my arms.

Wednesday 8th September 04.
I've known about the Chinese government's crackdown on *Falun Gong*, for a while. It's a meditation practice and philosophy, which appears to be a bit like *Tai Chi,* in that it has both a physical and contemplative aspect. Half of the leaflet Ioana gave me was promoting *Falun Gong* and the other half was asking for people to get involved in a campaign to free practitioners from unlawful imprisonment in China. I was drawn to an appealing image of a smiling mother holding up a robust looking baby for the photo. Two weeks later, the text tells us, both were dead. The mother's neck was broken and skull crushed following her appeal against the ban on *Falun Gong*. What totally horrified me was that, 'Her baby's ankles were badly bruised, his head dented and his nose full of blood. The examiner said the baby had been shackled and hung upside down'. The thought of the baby being tortured, perhaps in front of the mother, prior to her brutal murder, beggars belief. Who could do such a thing? And do they deserve to be called a human being?

Thursday 9th September 04.
Perhaps the French feminist Hélène Cixous was right when she suggested that women experience a more all-over body eroticism, whereas men are more interested in penile sensation; which is a posh way of saying that men are focussed on their nobs. Well, Robert is, anyway… Women desire sensual experience that encompasses their entire body – indeed, their entire being. Most men are too lazy to provide this. That's not to say that men are incapable of eroticism or sensuality – it's just a difference in emphasis. Men get so much pleasure from straightforward foreplayless penetrative sex that they forget that often this just doesn't do it for the

women. Can we reconcile these profound physiological and psychological differences?
I picked up a men's magazine recently at my local spa and flicked it open to a survey which suggested that 75% of women can orgasm during penetrative sex after 20 minutes of foreplay; this included licking, stroking, and, if enjoyed, bottom smacking – *only 20 minutes* – guys you can do this! So, as long as we are warmed up, the man can do his penetrative thing *and* make us happy was the message.
Personally, I like my inner-thighs and bottom to be stroked, licked or squeezed. Don't you? But if your man isn't interested how can you get him to realise that this bodily appreciation is sexier than going straight in for the clitoris? I guess I should own this problem. Having asked my partner to squeeze my arse at least *five thousand times*, it feels like, so what should I do when he frequently fails to do this? Send suggestions on a post-card please.

Friday 10th September 04.
Esmie is in hospital again. They thought she had meningitis and then viral encephalitis. Robert is just getting short text messages from Patrick so we don't really know what's going on. Encephalitis is an inflammation of the substance of the brain, and I imagine very, very, serious.

Saturday 11th September 04.
Viral encephalitis is very serious. A group of viruses, called enteroviruses, migrate, via blood, to the brain where they multiply. The immune system response causes the brain to swell. Permanent brain damage is a risk. The list of symptoms sounds pretty horrific and includes vomiting, confusion, seizures, paralysis and coma - poor little Esmie.

Sunday 12th September 04.
When 9/11 happened it haunted people's consciousness. Even those of us who missed the breathtakingly audacious terrorist attacks as they were happening heard broadcasts of the last conversations of those trapped in the burning building, saw photographs, listened to survivor's stories, and watched the footage of the planes fly into the Twin Towers as it was endlessly repeated. An event of similar magnitude has happened this

week. I deliberately didn't watch the news coverage but nevertheless what happened haunts my consciousness in a way that prevents my writing about anything else. I'm referring to the Muslim fundamentalist siege of the school in Beslan, Russia. To appreciate the horror you have know that when Russian troops stormed the building the terrorists began to mow down the children, others were burnt to death, some must have been killed in the cross-fire, or blown up by grenades. Hundreds were massacred.

I picked up Peter Conrad's critique of the media coverage of the event and now I can't get this picture out of my mind of the little girl who was literally blown out to safety by an explosion: 'rocketed to safety', to use his phrase. In the next frame of the three photographs he describes, 'she picks herself up and – wretchedly skinny, stripped, with scratched and bruised legs – climbs back in to the building.' The third photo shows the burning gym where the hostages were gathered. His comment, 'blown free, the anonymous child returns in time to die.' This little child too disorientated to run for freedom – to run for her life, turning the wrong way, haunts me.

Monday 13th September 04.

My new term-time routine has me coming home on most Mondays (rather than sleeping over near the University to get more hours in). When I arrived, both children launched themselves into my arms with screams of "huggie!" and "cuddle!". I had to keep taking turns to give them bear hugs until they were sated.

Later, I snuggled up with Eilish in her big double bed for stories; after stories we tell each other about our day: with three nice things and three not-so-nice, or horrible things, that happened to us. We've been doing the 'three things' since Eilish started school when it used to be really hard-work getting her to converse about her day at all. It used to be her who told three things, but now she insists on my reciprocating. And what are most joyous highlights of every day? Always, little insignificant moments, so insignificant I realise I've not generally even been recording them in this diary: the moment when Emile says, "mummy, I like you" in a slow and serious manner as though I'm not already aware of the fact, or the many infantile manifestations of gratuitous affection, so fleetingly bestowed, or the feeling of Eilish's soft warm little body in my arms – that's the one mums always mention. So many highlights, and I must choose only three. And what is all this? I guess it's happiness…

Tuesday 14th September 04.
In bed this evening, Eilish chose Babette Cole's *Mummy Laid an Egg* for her nightly reading practice. It's a wonderfully illustrated book about the 'facts of life'. It is slightly simplified with eggs inside "mummy's tummy", and "seeds" instead of sperm, but it's still very good. Anyway, after reading it Eilish turned to me and said, "you must thank the sperm that made me". "After all", she continued, "I might have turned out like X [horrible girl at school] if it had been a different sperm". I think she meant 'sperm donor'. I question her biological determinism, but thought her gratitude was endearing.

Wednesday 15th September 04.
I am working part-time now – did I tell you? This morning I sat in the sunshine in our garden while Emile pottered about. He picked the first apple to be harvested from a tree I had planted. Actually, he bent the bough of the tree towards himself and bit into the apple whilst it was still on the branch. "Not bad", was his pronouncement. I don't suppose it will give him the knowledge of the Gods, but it was great to see him eat something I planted…

Thursday 16th September 04.
Esmie is out of hospital and is 'fine'. I asked, "How do they know she is fine?", and Robert shrugged. How do you know if a newborn baby is brain damaged or not?

Saturday 18th September 04.
There was a withering review of Anne Enright's *Making Babies* in *Private Eye* this week. The book is 'affirmative goo' and 'she thinks she's the bee's knees' for having had a baby, it says. Have the reviewer and I read the same book, I wonder? Is he confusing some other text for the witty, iconoclastic, and self-depreciating book I've just enjoyed? And he doesn't even come out into the open – this is a nasty, malicious, anonymous

review. 'Stop drivelling and drooling. That's the baby's job', is the advice for those wishing to discuss motherhood. It's a good line, but utterly unjust. I liked Enright's book, which wasn't at all self-righteous because, *unlike* many other texts, it was positive about motherhood. The reviewer suggests that the market is already crowded by 'post-feminist reclamations of the moral right to motherhood' – not so! It's crowded by books claiming a moral right *not* to enjoy motherhood, or, rather, challenging the blithe assumption that we automatically will. These women writers grow into motherhood slowly and painfully; they *learn* to enjoy it with difficulty, and they mourn their old freedoms. They are not women who worked long shifts in a factory, for whom the experience of looking after a baby is a blessed relief from that toil and monotony; these are women who has nice life styles, nice apartments, nice friends, nice jobs – probably freelance… Indeed, I have wanted to slap writers such as Rachael Cusk for their joylessness, and their guilt-ridden anxiety. Will my baby be traumatised for life if I leave him with my mother for an evening? No, he'll be absolutely fine - stop torturing yourself, you daft cow! Sorry about that; I don't know what came over me!

The new writing is a more complex depiction of motherhood; it's a portrayal of adjustment. But the reviewer clearly hasn't read the books. I suppose it's not surprising to find men ready to depreciate a woman's enjoyment of her children.

Sunday 19th September 04.

"Readers might feel cheated if you don't get pregnant at the end", a writer friend suggests. "Perhaps you should keep writing it until you get pregnant", she offers. "But I'm beginning to think I will never get pregnant", I reply. Nevertheless, she urges me to keep writing.

Monday 20th September 04.

Trying to conceive is a limbo state. I've just seen a two-year fixed-contract research fellowship advertised at a good university. I feel ready for a change. I'd like to apply but if I get pregnant on such a short project that could really mess up their research schedule and without a good reference at the end I could end up unemployed. When should I simply start getting on with my life? When do you give up trying to have a baby?

Tuesday 21st September 04.

I worked late at the office. I didn't manage to get all my work done even so and I wonder how working part-time is going to be – whether I'll be seen as the departmental slacker. And what will happen when I get my piles of marking and tight marking deadlines? Will I be allowed to claim back my overtime? Or will other people take on some of the marking? Or will I, as I suspect, simply be expected to put in the extra hours?

So as I say, I worked late at the office so only got to spend a few minutes with Eilish before her lights off time. I hate it when I get stuck in traffic and miss being able to put her to bed. Emile, on the other hand, is now up to 9.30pm every night so I get to sing him songs in his cot and stroke his little head and cuddle him.

Even though we had a massive row on Sunday, I felt tender towards Robert as we put Emile to bed together.

Saturday 25th September 04.

Saturday night is Robert and my night out together – our special time together. His conversational opener, as we sit down with our drinks in the theatre bar, is "Esmie's dead".

He has been fretting, "I'm sure she's dead because the only time Patrick didn't answer his phone before was when she was critically ill in hospital and I've been texting him and he hasn't answered…" I suppose this explains why he has been high-strung and moody. I take a rational approach, "he's knackered and preoccupied, that's all", I retort. "Esmie's not sleeping for five hour stretches like Emile did…" But I feel for him and suggest he sends a text saying he's worrying, which he does. Then we see a play and continue with our lives…

Sunday 26th September 04.

Patrick texted Robert to say he is "too tired to live" but is otherwise fine. I use this as an opportunity to tease Robert about his pessimistic nature, "You killed off Esmie…you must get a grip…" His mood palpably improves.

Monday 27th September 04.

I stayed overnight with my friends Sarah and John who have a little boy,

Vandon, who I guess must be about two by now. He wakes up in the night and shuffles whining down the corridor to their bed. Once in he must be cuddled to sleep by Sarah before she can slink out to the spare room to get some space and sleep. I remember Eilish climbing out of her cot at about the same age – throwing herself onto a hard floor, opening her door, walking in the dark along a corridor, opening my door and then climbing into my bed. She was remarkably stubborn, and I feared real injury from the cot escapes, so in the end I just continued to sleep with her… The intimacy of sleeping with a baby is lovely but they don't adjust easily to sleeping alone it seems. Emile only slept in my bed for the first few weeks; then I had him in a Moses basket next to the bed, and now he goes to sleep in his cot quite uncomplainingly after our little bedtime rituals. He never thinks of climbing out. He hasn't the deep longing for my body that she had.

Wednesday 29th September 04.

Robert shouted, no, in fact, Robert screamed, because Eilish came downstairs and asked me to draw the curtains in her room five minutes after her bedtime. There was a chink in the curtains creating ominous shadows on the wall of her room. "I'm sick of this fucking bullshit…" Actually, it was the first time she'd disturbed us after her bedtime for yonks – many, many months. And so what if a seven year old is a little afraid at bedtime from time to time…? At her age I remember I believed that the furniture moved about after dark – a peculiar anthropomorphism which had me creeping fearfully past wardrobes expecting them to leap out at me… As I lay in my bed in the gloom, I thought the dancing master, in the picture by Degas, which hung on my bedroom wall, waved his cane – *I could see it*. I can remember being frightened to be on my own at night-time. Eilish is a sweet little girl and I wonder why my partner is screaming like a mad person at her? What have I done to create this situation? I hadn't irritated him by being late…When I tried to talk to him he said I was "terrified to discipline her". But he is so off the mark here. Why should I want to discipline her for her childish fears – fears I remember so well myself? I want her to feel happy. I want to comfort her. I want her to feel safe.

And why would he want to send a sobbing child to bed (sobbing only after he's roared at her) to lie distressed and fearful in the dark? And how could he expect me as her mother to tolerate that? What kind of man is he? I fear for my children with this man and his sadistic impulses, his harsh ideas about discipline, and lack of warmth. I seem to have everything and yet it is slipping away from me – my job, this lovely house which I imagine walking out of with only a few bags and my children…

Thursday 30th September 04.
I'm not sure I'll be having conception sex with Robert tonight. It's day fourteen so we should be having sex, but I feel too bloody angry after his bad behaviour last night.

Friday 1st October 04.
Well perhaps the reader will feel cheated. The only new baby in this book, which is nearing its end, is Esmie who belongs to friends of Robert's who I hardly know; I've only actually met them once so, of course, I feel emotionally remote from their drama, except vicariously via Robert's anxiety about the whole experience. But it looks as though Esmie is fine and that they'll visit soon, then I'll get to hold her and she'll seem real to me at last.

Monday 4th October 04.
Everybody's family is difficult - are there any problem free families out there? Anyway, this little vignette will perhaps give a taste of our mealtime tensions. Robert's parents, Jacquie and Rumy, took us to *Candytown*: a nice, local, child tolerant Chinese restaurant with terrible decor; It should have been relaxing. I found myself sandwiched between them, at a round-table, as Rumy started to tell me about Parsi-Indian friends of his who have moved to Sweden and who are having trouble finding husbands for their three daughters. The daughters are all in their late thirties and are trained doctors; and this is the problem, of course, that they are highly trained professionals. It is taboo to the Parsi culture that they might marry men who are not equivalently trained. Rumy may have used the words, "top quality" – "they need husbands who are top quality". Also, unlike many other cultural groups, such as Pakistani Muslims, in Parsi culture the husband joins their new wife's family. Anyway, I find all

this fascinating; I am an amateur anthropologist finding out about their, to me, very foreign cultures. Of course, this isn't just a Parsi problem as high achieving women find it difficult to find comparable partners in general, as Hewlett's research, which I discussed earlier, illustrated. Thus, finding three nice, high-powered Parsi-Indian professional husbands willing to relocate to Sweden for these perhaps-too-old-to-have-babies Parsi doctors was proving to be impossible! This was intriguing and I was asking whether the parents would consider allowing them to marry 'out' as attracting a Swedish high-powered professional might prove a less insuperable possibility, when Jacquie chipped in with, "it's like the middle-ages isn't it"? Then she added, "The way, they treat women: it's appalling", in case I had failed to register her distain. She exuded contempt for all this Parsi nonsense. I was piggy in the middle. On the one hand, I didn't want to get drawn in to a critique of the treatment of women in traditional Parsi circles; I *can* see the value of remaining part of a community and retaining that community's support. It's not my community and it's not how I'd want to live but I can respect other ways of organising things. Nor, on the other hand, did I want to be seen to be snubbing Jacquie by not responding to her point. After all, she was appealing to me for support as a feminist. Of course I believe women must be free to choose their husbands if they so wish and that communities who punish or otherwise reject women for so doing are reprehensible; however, I don't think traditional ways of doing things are wrong *per se.* Then one of those uneasy silences ensued, so characteristic of eating with his family, but fortunately the children then dominated our attention.

Wednesday 8th October 04.

I was having lunch with a friend in a little Italian restaurant and a very loud woman picked up her baby held it aloft and pronounced for all to hear in a sing-song voice, "you've done an poo, yooov'e done a poo-poo, yes, you have - yooov'e done a *great big poo-poo*. I can smell it...." And so forth. She proceeded to repeatedly and ostentatiously sniff the offending bottom whist bleating on in the aforementioned manner. I imagine I wasn't the only person who wanted to yell, "we don't all want to think about your baby's shit while we're eating", or "get a life!" or, "shut up moron!". Now I am reminded why mothers sometimes get a bad press...

Friday 10th October 04.
After my Well Woman check up it seems I'm quite healthy (though I've got to see an ophthalmologist); it's nice to know that I'm not about to die on my kids!

Monday 11th October 04.
I was willing to be the primary wage earner but Robert has consistently refused to move. When we met I earned more than him, and I still do pro-rata. Occasionally, I've been audacious enough to dangle a research fellowship in Sydney under his nose or to suggest that Edinburgh isn't a million miles away. I've seen lovely, lovely jobs for which I'd have stood a chance drift way. I've felt sorry for myself, frustrated, angry, and wistful in turns; I have endured this silently. Today, after I gave up my lunch break to do our vegetable shopping at PAKS food store, as is my custom on Mondays, I trudged in wearily from working late in the office, again, to receive a lecture from Robert about how I should have bought a 10 litre sack of Basmati rice, rather than a 20 litre sack – I *don't think* about our budget he asserted, and he just wouldn't drop it; I remember how nice it was to handle my own money on my own and, funny this, I always had enough money for food and I never had to think about whether to buy a big or small sack of something; why this is really galling is because Robert is a bad shopper – he buys expensive things in small quantities, uses our very expensive local shops, and the fancy cooking he likes to do costs us per meal at least three times that of my more simple fare; yet I get the bloody lecture, and I endure it *silently*...

Tuesday 12th October 2004.
My life is crazy. The photocopiers at work aren't working and packs of students are wandering around looking for their lectures which have been rescheduled or moved to another venue; my colleagues are cranky and I wear a *I'm too busy to talk to you* expression on my face; it's surprisingly effective. At home things are no better as there are squirrels in our loft space requiring inhumane eviction – nobody thinks me prodding the nest with a broom will be sufficient; then there's building work required to stop more squirrels getting back in. Eilish has got nits again! I may have nits; I haven't had time to check, but perhaps my head only itches when I think

about hers… The car tax needs renewing and I happen to know there is no money left in our joint account to cover this, or the squirrels. Robert decided to force-feed Emile his spaghetti last night just to remind me that he is a fundamentally unreasonable person. I couldn't enjoy giving Eilish her bath or starting her stories at all because I could hear was Robert shouting and Emile crying. After what seemed like an eternity, but was actually about twenty minutes, I went downstairs and said calmly that it's impossible to force-feed a baby, that it's not thought to be good practice by anyone, and that the noise of Emile crying was upsetting me. Robert stomped out of the house. Must add that to my list of things to do: *leave husband.*

Wednesday 13th October 04.
I didn't sleep well last night, not because of the tension yesterday but because I dreamt about Emile dying on the operating table; I have done a very good job of screening out all thoughts of his impending surgery but the event is forcing its way into my consciousness now.

Thursday 14th October 04.
Emile announced, "I'm feeling happy today", and he is - such a happy little baby, and I wonder if he'll feel betrayed by us when he lies in hospital in pain tomorrow not understanding what's going on, yet I'll be so relieved to experience his anger and resentment, to know that now it's over, that he is safe.
I meant to take him swimming this morning, but I forgot; he loves it and he'll not be able to go for ages now because of the stitches, and I feel *guilty* now because I forgot that I'd meant to take him, but when I woke up this morning I just had this vague sense that there was something I was *meant* to do; you know what it's like, but there was nothing written in my diary, and I only remembered about the idea of taking him swimming when I thought about his operation again, and, as I say, now I feel guilty, which I know is irrational because I didn't tell Emile he was going swimming, and even if I had told him he'd have forgotten because he only has a toddler's memory.

Friday 15th October 04.

Before, I was awash with hormones. Then I got pregnant again and miscarried so that kept the chemical cocktail boosted. Yesterday, I realised that I no longer feel 'broody' in that palpable way anymore; that deep longing seems to have subsided within me. Perhaps trying to have a baby has been a sort of mourning process for the baby I lost, and now I feel resolved. I have two gorgeous children and that will be enough for me. It may have to be. I am edging slowly, so slowly, towards acceptance of the fact that I shall not have a third child.

***

Today is the day for his surgery. I am waiting for Emile to wake. We let him sleep late so he won't get too hungry, and cranky, before his operation; because he's having general anaesthetic he can have only water and apple juice, so we were tactical and kept him up late last night, and gave him a late supper. Hopefully, he won't be screaming for food by the time we get him to the operating table.

I just heard him stir and must go; the day I have feared has just begun.

Saturday 17th October 04.

Yesterday was a *long day*. We both were dreading him going under the general anaesthetic. The late supper worked and, miraculously, he didn't even ask for food before his operation. He was allowed apple juice at 10.30 a.m. and that filled up his tummy. He played in the playroom and, apart from one authoritarian nurse irritating me, the day went smoothly. The consultant came and explained the procedure again to us, in case we'd forgotten, I suppose. Then it was just a question of waiting until his 2.00pm slot. Unfortunately, hospital policy only allowed one of us into the pre-operative anaesthesia room. Why the hospital should want to torture parents in this way, I have no idea. The room had a hospital bed in it and lots of machines and three members of staff in it: the anaesthetist; a trainee anaesthetist, and a nurse (the authoritarian one). On the wall was a mural with lots of animals, but on closer inspection they were all injured: the mother sow had a dressed wound on her back, and so forth. At first he clung on to me like a baby monkey. I had to bribe him with the promise of a polo-mint if he'd "lie nicely" on the bed.

I had to distract him with a book that played tunes while they fitted a catheter and administered the first dose of general anaesthetic (I actually sang *Twinkle, Twinkle Little Star*, his favourite bed-time song. What a betrayal!). The injection rendered him unconscious almost immediately. Then a mask was popped onto his face and he was wheeled off into the surgery and I was left standing, feeling blank, knowing that this could be the last time I'd see him alive.

This time I didn't cry. Perhaps it was because Eilish had had general anaesthetic earlier in the year and I'd faced the possibility of the death of a child back then; perhaps that experience had anaesthetised my own feelings. It's Robert who's been doing the weeping in the last twenty-four hours, though a single tear glided down my cheek late last night I admit as I tried to sleep. Or perhaps, to view my experience more positively, I have become slightly more rational. When I visited Graham, (my friend now living in Amsterdam), when he was in hospital, I could hardly to bear to be there – my feelings of claustrophobia were overwhelming. I hate hospitals. I must have been a dull and unsatisfactory visitor sitting squeamish and squirming and leaving after a very short visit consisting mainly of me moaning about how much I detest hospitals.

A few months ago, when Eilish was in hospital I wept and I almost passed-out when she had her catheter inserted; the nurse has to stop what she was doing to get *me* a glass of water. I remember Eilish saying, "mummy don't cry". In Accident and Emergency and in the pre-operative anaesthesia room I felt nauseous. I was tense *all the time*.

On this occasion, I only almost passed-out once, and this was after Emile's surgery when, back on his ward, I was drawn to a little child, around Eilish's age, having what I suppose was a blood transfusion. There was this bag of blood attached to the side of her bed and it kept filling up, and I kept looking at it. Her bed was in front of me; I couldn't help but see it. And every time I looked at it I felt sick and wanted to run away. But I couldn't leave because there in front of me was Emile: languid on the hospital bed, groggy with morphine, white faced, disorientated, fragile; so I was trapped. I tried not to glance at the bag of blood but it seemed to draw me back. The bag of blood haunted my consciousness; I couldn't not look at it. Emile clung on to me, and there I was suspended in a moment which seemed to last forever. I stroked Emile's hot forehead; I looked at the machines: the tubes and saline drips, and at the bag of blood. Yes, it was filling up, but very very slowly. Surely, if it were a blood transfusion it would be filling up more quickly? Are transfusions really that slow? But what else can it be? I am ignorant; I am too ignorant.

I turn from the bag of blood to watch the emaciated little girl in the other corner of the room. She is Emile's age and I think she is dying of something. Shall I ask the mother, "Hi, what's wrong with your little girl?" Hospital wards are weird places, which force you into unwanted relationships with others immediately. No, I don't need to know what's killing her child. I don't need them in my life at all. The little girl almost chokes at one point, so I cannot not be aware of her drama. A nurse is summoned. I take furtive glances at her to relieve the boredom: now she is taking her inhaler, now some medicine, now she is drinking, now gagging. Her mother disappears for several minutes and returns with a poke of chips. The little girl clamours for a chip but is told that they are too indigestible for her tummy. I wonder what illness she has which would make a potato taboo. She is so painfully thin she looks in need of some potatoes.

I try not to think about them. The little girl with the bag of blood had been playing with Emile earlier though, in a big-sisterly kind of way; I guess that's why I care about her. Now she is weeping from her pain and I wonder, as I walk past her bed on my way to the loo, whether I should acknowledge her or not: I could nod or smile. I take a furtive glance but she is too absorbed now in her suffering to notice me.

And eventually, after seeing the consultant again and filling in forms and waiting for a nurse to dress his wounds and remove the catheter inserted into his wrist, we are walking home in the cool night air. Emile is not going to die; he's not going to die today, at least.

When we get home, I let Eilish downstairs from bed to give Emile the beautiful get well card she'd made for him and Robert harshly barks at me for letting her and I lose it entirely and rant that he is a bullying tyrant and that I want him out of my life.

Sunday 18th October 04.

Well it's time to get serious about motherhood. No I don't mean I'm considering having IVF, there are moments when I feel tempted but these are brief.

Motherhood kills. Hundreds of thousands of women are dying needlessly each year because of inadequate, or non-existent, sexual and reproductive heath services. Here are a few sobering statistics: an estimated 201 million women globally would like to use contraception but are unable to get access to it (this is about one in seven women of reproductive age in the developing world). Every minute in the world someone is dying of a pregnancy-related cause. Every year 529,000 women die from pregnancy related causes – imagine the Titanic filled with pregnant women sinking every single day of the year. And, of course, if the mothers die their existing children are at risk. Where is the most dangerous place to have a baby? In sub-Saharan Africa 1 in 16 women die from a complication related to pregnancy or in childbirth. What is sexual and reproductive health? One health worker in Kenya put it like this: 'I would say that a packet of [contraceptive] pills is an entry point to giving the woman health education on issues of nutrition, breast-feeding, sexually transmitted diseases and HIV/Aids.' So, sexual and reproductive health (SRH) is wide-ranging; it includes the provision of obstetric care and abortion. Some organisations also work against practices such as female genital mutilation. In Kenya, abortion is illegal, and the maternal death rate is 871 deaths per 100,00 births, and up to 54% of these deaths are thought to be the result of unsafe abortion. Not surprisingly, many organisations providing SRH want to be able to offer safe abortions to women who need them as part of their services.

Unfortunately, the Bush administration's domestic agenda: civil rights for foetuses and reduced access to abortion has become enshrined in international policy, channelling millions of dollars away from SRH for women in the third world. Basically, the Bush administration has imposed conditions on foreign aid and now prohibits international organisations from providing abortion or abortion advice or to lobby their own governments to legalise abortion. One organisation alone, The United Nations Population Fund, lost $34 million dollars destined for SRH work in 120 countries. Well, you get the picture. The largest single donor of world aid, the U.S., has greatly curtailed its funding of SRH aid and seeks to 'gag' organisations which promote safe abortion practices. Meanwhile, the quality of life for millions of women, unable to control their fertility, remains precarious. As Sue George puts it: '…when a man in the developed world wants a condom, he simply buys one. It is a very different situation from that faced by men in sub-Saharan Africa. Statistics from the United Nations Population Fund (UNFPA) show that if the available supply in the region was evenly distributed, then each man would receive just three a year. That's not a great deal of help in preventing sexually transmitted infections (including HIV, which has wreaked havoc across that continent) or pregnancy'. When a poor woman in a poor county gets pregnant her life is at risk.

Sunday 24th October 04.

This week has seen an unedifying skirmish in the press about whether babies are boring or not. The controversial and widely reviled author, Anna Pasternak has come out as feeling 'trapped, and, frankly bored' by motherhood. She's had lots of media attention for her trivial remarks. There is a peculiar riposte in *The Observer*, though whether or not it is properly a refutation is open to question because at one point the author, Viv Groskop, seems to think it's not surprising that women who are 'selfish' enough to develop a range of interests and a career prior to motherhood might find it boring. She rants about mothers leaving motherhood so late they are 'too old to really enjoy it'. Indeed, 'The longer you wait the more selfish you become' and, what's more, 'according to Mother Nature after the age of 35 you are just too old to be having your first baby.' After this grotesque, utterly unjustifiable, ageism the author makes one useful point about how women *have* to postpone motherhood if they are ambitious. The 'later first pregnancy… is a solution that permits women into the world of work and education on male terms – …they [must] delay having a child for as long as possible and then pretend they don't really have one… it is culturally unacceptable – and professionally impossible – for women to have children earlier.' Well, how about a bit of sympathy for your older sisters then, Viv? And isn't all this 'work-life balance' stuff supposed to challenge both our status as honorary men (while we are childless) and provoke men to think about parenting their children on an equal basis? They are missing out on what could become the most meaningful bit of their lives. Isn't that the point of 'work life balance': that men prioritise their families more too?

Thursday 4th November 04.

There's been a gap in this diary because my computer was stolen. We were burgled. I'm writing on Eilish's little lap-top, having bought some software as mine was stolen, and it feels really weird: I miss my spacious key board, big screen, and mouse. But the absence of a computer has meant that I've spent an unprecedented amount of time with the children. And that's the paradox of this book: it takes me away from them. I do want to set the record straight about a minor point. Well, perhaps it's not so insignificant. In March, I envisaged a scene (Thursday 13th March 2003., to be precise), in which I imagined Eilish, Emile and me in the garden with a new-born baby. I imagined Emile ranging into the flowerbeds and tearing up clumps of plants. His older sister was depicted as retrieving him repeatedly, patiently, but too roughly, so that he ended up screaming and complaining. I saw myself as tense and alert. Above all, I depicted us as unable to do anything because Emile would disrupt any complex game we attempted to play; I envisaged a frustrating situation. It was a negative picture of motherhood evoked by anxiety and uncertainty about how I'd cope with more babies. But actually, it has not been like that. Of course there is no new born evoking jealousy in her older siblings, but Emile showed no propensity to wreck the garden this summer. Indeed, he was able to potter about in a rather self-contained way for hours at a time. Eilish remains attention-seeking – why, oh why? I wish I knew, but even she relaxes a bit outside. Now, it is cold and our forays into the garden are sporadic, and I miss that unanticipated relaxed freedom. (Indeed, if it were mid-summer I'd be out there now and not typing on a p.c.).

Imagine, instead of the earlier scene, Emile playing with his sand pit: he picks up a spade full of sand and with great concentration steps out of the sandpit. He holds the spade in front of him taking great care not to spill a drop; then, having reached his desired spot at a bit of dry-stone walling on the other side of the garden, he flings it into the air! And then he does it all over again. Eilish is doing some sort of imaginative play: she is a restaurateur asking what I fancy from the menu, then rushing off to make it with twigs and stones as in her schema the *maitre d* is also the wine waitress, and cook; or perhaps she's off with her imaginary friends in fairy-land (which doesn't involve me). Now Emile is sitting in his plastic car imaging going somewhere and shuffling it across the lawn with his feet. Visualize me reading a book, between interruptions to make orders from the menus, and the leaves turning burnt umber, yellow and many hues of red. Days pass like this. We are relaxed and happy together. If I'd had a new-born baby on my lap it would have been like that too. Robert is absent from the picture though – he doesn't like the garden. He doesn't really like being outside at all. He may be absent from our future (mine and the children's) and I am beginning to think that will be okay. My desire for a third child is being displaced by a wistful sadness.

Friday 5th November 04.
"*Remember, Remember the 5th of November,*
Gunpowder, treason and plot,
There is no reason why gun- powder treason,
Should ever be forgot".

Like it or not, having children makes you engage with a larger reality – strange though it might be. When I collected Eilish from Katie's house, after her "play-over", she was dancing in the garden, in Katie's clothes, with sparklers in both hands. The local pub offers a good fireworks display I'm told. Shall we go? I have a momentary flash-back of watching the fireworks from the roof of my flat in Edinburgh. I recall the concert and synchronised display, enjoyed with a bottle of wine and friends (a child-free past which was mourned when I first had Eilish). It is a very fleeting vision as I am eating home-made toffee and making polite conversation with Eilish's new best friend's parents. Both seem perfectly nice in an insipid way. Then I'm whisking her off to our bonfire and sparklers - they are too young to demand fireworks yet. Besides, there are bangs and crashes everywhere; we don't need to create our own. Robert, as he (symbolically and literally) hoses down our bonfire later says, "I'll make veggi-burgers and hot dogs next year", and then perhaps he catches a glimpse of my expression and adds, "If we're still together". I say something anodyne in reply. Last year he lounged on the sofa while I did bonfire night alone with the children (I find it hard to forgive that sort of domestic betrayal). The year before that he'd visited me in my cottage and been obliged to join in with the festivities I'd arranged with a friend and her son. He had seemed more promising then; nevertheless, my optimism is real. I hope we will be together this time next year eating hot dogs with the children, warmed by our bonfire.

Friday 12th November 2004.

Isobel came for a "sleepover". I like 'Izzy' and her parents; although, I've still no idea what Michael actually does for a living. Izzy says, "He works in Manchester". Anyway, he exudes charm and Eilish loves going to their house. I don't think he's a mafia boss or anything distasteful. I've only met the mother once (Izzy says she's a florist) but they entrust their daughter into my care and vice-versa. Izzy is a long-standing friend and even though she's moved school we are keeping in touch. She is very bright and funny though she likes to get her own way: I deal with this by saying that the guest gets to choose the activity; consequently, they don't argue about what to do as Eilish is concerned to be a good host.

Robert just won't be positive about Eilish at the moment. Even though Izzy whinged more than Eilish, was demanding and generally rather impolite, refused to eat the pasta sauce, refused to help me pack her bag at the end and was thoroughly "a little madam" as Robert put it, he still wouldn't acknowledge that Eilish is exceptionally well-behaved for her age (I want to make it clear to the reader that I consider Izzy's behaviour as quite typical for her age group and that I regard Robert's expectations as *unreasonable*). "Perhaps she's better behaved at home", he retorted. I have decided that it's time for a reality check and I am intending to invite all Eilish's best friends over for play sessions before Christmas so he can see what children of that age are really like.

Saturday 13th November 04.

The National mood is shifting. Tony Blair was on the radio saying that the school day doesn't correspond to working parent's lives and that he intends to offer pre-school and after-school provision on a universal basis. This sounds promising. He didn't mention nursery services though. My friend Sarah has worked out that following her maternity leave she'll be paying over 1,000 pounds per month in nursery fees, which is a bit stiff. I'll get my five free 2.5-hour sessions starting from January after Emile turns three; however, they will not be much help unless there is someone around to drop Emile off and pick him up. The opposition is advocating vouchers – they could be spent to pay a grandparent to baby sit, said a spokesman. I though this rather bizarre example as those who have grandparents to baby sit already have this, if you see what I mean. The three sets of grandparents relating to our children live in Stevenage, London and the Isle-of-Wight and cash incentives will have no impact on their willingness or availability.

Sunday 14th November 04.
My period started. We've been hitting the right days following the ovulation test. Although, we made a resolution sometime ago to give up trying-to-have-baby sex, and to just have sex when we feel like it, we haven't stuck to the resolve, such is our desire for me to conceive. Every time I have a period I feel gutted now.

Tuesday 16th November 04.
Do we know anyone able to offer some sperm, Robert was asked today. Launa has decided to have another baby and is on the look out for a sperm donor. She is just after the sperm – this would be a non-sexual liaison. She propositioned Robert at the nursery gate – not for his sperm, but for a friend's. She is nothing if not forward.

Wednesday 17th November 04.
Our regrets affect our children. What are my regrets, apart from the massive one of not having had more children? I wish I had properly mastered a foreign language and I wish I had learnt a musical instrument; consequently, and not unreasonably I feel, I'd like Eilish to do both. I also wish I'd travelled more, and that is still possible as I intend to take Eilish to at least one European country each year. No doubt, she'll be whinging about that soon: "Oh, God; not another of mummy's long weekends".
Anyway, because she forgot to give me the form, she didn't get the opportunity to start on a 'proper' instrument this year at school. Her school arranges music lessons and has a small number of flutes, clarinets, violins and key-boards for a few keen students. However, by the time I got the application form, which had languished in her bag for over a month (guilt, guilt why hadn't I checked?), they'd all been allocated. She'll have

to wait until September now. She says she is really keen but I imagine with the *reality* of *daily* practice playing a real instrument would soon lose its allure.

We were in the car at the time. Eilish shouted at me because she didn't want to go Music Playtime. She seems to sense my unexpressed desires and to thwart them: there is an emotional violence in this somehow. First she refused to speak French even though she was semi-fluent as a result of having had a string of French au-pairs. One day she simply refused to speak it. I feel terrible that she has forgotten it all now; it seems such a waste. She lost interest in her dance classes after just one term; that didn't bother me really as so many of the participants seemed so dreadfully *wannabe*. I was only there under duress. But now she's rejecting music which I care about and which was noted as her best subject in last year's school report. She says the recorder is "boring". Indeed, a few days ago she pronounced that reading was "boring". This was the ultimate rejection of her parent's values given Robert's obsessive interest in the mechanics of the English language as a linguist, and my own history of writing for publication as an academic. Fortunately, her friend, Izzy, was visiting at the time and forcefully confronted her. Izzy then proceeded to read several bedtime stories out-loud, which served to underline her point that reading is fun.

There is something perverse about Eilish. When I replied that I thought she should keep going to Music Play Time until they start musical instruments at school next year she burst into tears and wailed. Anyway, after being ratty with me, she announced that she now wants to go to back to the French breakfast club she used to attend, where they have croissants and jam and play games in French instead of Music Play Time. I certainly think she should try to do *something* in a sustained way.

I know what this is about: I *resent* the fact that my parents never seemed to have any aspirations for me, except the find a good husband and marry and have two kids variety which blighted many of my generations of girls. They discouraged me from doing all kinds of things, and only pushed typing lessons, as I recall. But are my aspirations for my daughter insidiously oppressive and destructive? Will she end up *resenting* me? "Mummy, you were always making me *do things*, when I just wanted to play..."

Thursday 18th November 04.
Emile had his post-operative check at the children's hospital today. After a mammoth wait in trying circumstances: a busy, crowded and noisy waiting room, the consultant had a quick look and pronounced that he was doing well. The testicle might "shrivel up" in the next six months due to insufficient blood supply but this is not dangerous, though he might decide to have prosthesis later on if this were to happen. The testicle is looking good though, he said, so that's unlikely. The final, hopefully final, appointment will be in May. After that, I don't want to see that children's hospital ever again.

Friday 19th November 04.
Graham is visiting from Amsterdam. He's a pianist but didn't start playing until he was eleven. He thinks seven is too young to start sustained practice with a musical instrument. I should relax. And no, he's not interested in donating sperm to Launa! Well, I had to ask.

Saturday 20th November 04.
Graham says Robert is "complex". Indeed, he says it is a slightly mincing way and tosses his hair, now long, when he drawls: "well, I think you are *eversooooo lucky* to have such a *complex* man in your life; I think he's *absolutely lovely*". He even calls him my "toy-boy". Graham isn't normally camp but he's got quite a flirty thing going with Robert: He even ruffles his hair! And Robert responds and gets quite boyish and playful. One of the things I most dislike about Robert is that he is too often the humourless, strutting patriarch, keeping us all in line and spoiling the atmosphere, the *joie de vivre*. Yes, there is water on the bathroom floor but we are all enjoying ourselves… he kills our fun. Yet he's so charming when he relaxes so I feel quite envious that Graham has this knack of bringing out this best side of his personality.

Thursday 25th November 04.
Anyway, part of Robert's lovely complexity is his new obsession that I not see his flaccid penis. He gets possessed with doing things a certain way and then he seems to *have* to do it like that and then it shifts but in the same way: to something new but something he seems to *have* to do again.

He used to have an obsession with me kneeling and then he'd slide under my legs so that I was effectively sitting on his face, but with me bearing my weight, but I really can't remember the last time we did that now...We have been having quite a lot of sex and obviously some of it at times when we'd probably not have bothered because of trying to conceive. Robert likes to stroke me while I lay on the bed or for us to stand up kissing and fondling prior to getting down to things. I think it helps him quiet his mind. A few months ago he asked me to oil him; "baba, will you oil me now", has become a frequent refrain. At which point he pulls off his boxer shorts and stands in front of me – and there is it: his manhood in all its glory, arching skywards slightly. I don't know why he gets me to oil him so often: something to do with getting it so hard he can't lose the erection later on. I have to warm baby oil on my hands and stoke his balls and penis. I sit on the bed and he stands, so I'm looking up at his chunky hairy body, which I adore. It's by candle-light, and it would be very, very sexy if he didn't ask me to do it quite so bloody often.

Really good sex is spontaneous, passionate and varied. Robert is becoming gradually more passionate and less controlled – he's started doing this thing where he nuzzles and stiffs my body; it's quite animalistic and I really like it. Trying to conceive a baby has distracted us from our straightforward enjoyment of sex. Robert used to engage in far more foreplay in the past, but now the goal is "getting seed in me" and it feels as though he's in a hurry to achieve this aim. He does give me orgasms but, again, it often feels as though he's in a hurry. He's got into the habit.

Friday 26th November 04.

It's day fourteen of my fertility cycle and my Clearblue ovulation test showed no surge, indicating that I'm not ovulating yet, but am I ovulating at all? That's what I want to find out. No ovulation means we don't have to have sex tonight but we might anyway.

Saturday 27th November 04.

No surge as expected. My last detected surge was on day fifteen of my cycle so I feel disappointed.

Sunday 28th November 04.
No surge again; a late ovulation then? I groan inwardly at the thought that I am now on the cusp of menopause.

Monday 29th November 04.
No surge again. Do I have a slightly masochistic streak to keep putting myself through this?

Tuesday 30th November 04.
A colleague and I got chatting about how we enjoy being parents and I ended up saying I wouldn't mind one more. Very British, really: "I wouldn't mind having one more". No mention of all the existential pain involved, of course.

Wednesday 1st December 04.
She has a vision in her mind of picking up her new born infant by her ankles, swinging her round in the air and dashing her head against a wall. The baby's head explodes on impact and the brains and blood splatter the wall. This is the vision she has. Sometimes it is a waking vision. She is pushing the buggy along the street, on some ordinary shopping errand, and the image invades her consciousness; she shoos away the thoughts but they return later in a dream. She wakes in a state of panic, gulping for air. It is the same image over and over again. It is the same violent impulse over and over again. She is the woman in the vision. The baby is hers. Is she mad? Is she a danger to her offspring? The thought horrifies her. She feels she wants to keep her baby safe. Above all else this is what she feels, so why does she have this repeating image of murder in her mind? Perhaps as compensation for the vision she watches her baby with special vigilance.
Her other recurring nightmare is the converse, or it appears to be; she is usually on a ship (though it is occasionally an aeroplane crash landed into water) and they are drowning and she must get out of the enclosed space and she must survive. Above all, she must save her baby. But the baby is no longer newborn; indeed, the baby is now a large heavy toddler and she is swimming and struggling. She is an excellent swimmer and a strong woman yet the weight of the toddler is pulling her down, pulling her

down, but she won't let go: she will drown first. And she does, she drowns, all the time trying to save the baby. Finally, the water fills her lungs and she starts to drown rather than let go of her infant. And it is while she is dying she wakes: bolt upright in bed, drenched in sweat, gulping for air and crying out. Why would she sacrifice herself for something so partially formed? Or perhaps she feels engulfed by motherhood, swallowed up by it as if it's the sea – a sea of mothering? Is she mad?

I remember my old self. What does it mean that I no longer have these nightmares? It has taken me a long time to feel at ease with being a mother.

Thursday 2nd December 04.

Robert has already calculated that I'm likely to be ovulating on Christmas Day and I think he's a bit gutted, as he really wanted to gorge himself but won't be able to have sex if he eats too much!

Wednesday 8th December 04.

My period started early and Robert was pleased because it means all our conception sex will be done before Christmas Eve and then he can eat and drink to excess without having to worry about his erection!

Thursday 9th December 04.

He was adamant about going this morning. "Emile, you'd like to come shopping with mummy" I'd try. "No, I want swimming" he'd reply. He's suddenly developed a memory which is rather inconvenient. I made several other attempts, "wouldn't you like to see the toy trains in the shopping centre?" Which was answered with a resolute, "I want swimming". Yesterday, I'd said, "tomorrow we can go shopping or swimming together". I was already in my costume in the changing rooms when Emile refused to undress. I explained that he wouldn't be allowed into the pool with his clothes on. He shrieked when I tried to take them off. The two older ladies in the changing room both had a go at persuading him what fun it would be to put his trunks on and swim. It ended up being quite a funny scene with us all trying to reason with him and jolly him along. He was standing with arms crossed, shaking his head, frowning and pouting (looking very serious, yet incredibly cute: like a disgruntled angel). Eventually, when I described the special floats, he got excited and capitulated.

Thursday 16th December 04.
Bizarrely, he did precisely the same thing again this week – getting to the changing rooms and then refusing to undress, though he loved it once we were in the water and spent a lot of time just floating. I wonder if he felt uncomfortable undressing in front of the strange ladies? I'll have to try the little changing cubicle next time.

Friday 17th December 04.
I forgot to set my alarm clock, overslept and missed Eilish's school play on at 9.15am. "It's about Italy" she'd told me, "and we sing *Christmas Tree, Oh Christmas Tree* in German…" I was actually quite curious to see what peculiar multi-cultural mix they'd come up with. She'll be very upset when she realises I didn't make it… Needless to say, this has spoilt my day!

***

I took Eilish out for ice cream after school to make up for oversleeping and missing her play. She was actually very relaxed about it. I guess she got used to me not being there when I worked full-time.

Saturday 18th December 04.
Robert's cousin, Farzad, is lonely doing work experience in Hammersmith says Rumy, and will we take him in for Christmas? Of course, there is no question of saying no, and, besides, I liked Farzad when I met him at Katherine's Parsi wedding feast, before her marriage. Eilish's oft repeated refrain, "Why do Indians get to wear all the best clothes?" was mainly prompted that day by Farzad's sister and mother in their flowing saris. I'm looking forward to all the feast food, especially the Indian curries which Robert will make.

Sunday 19th December 04.
I intend to launch myself into the festive season with abandon so I don't think I'll be making any more diary entries until after Christmas. Wish me luck.

Wednesday 29th December 04.

Christmas went well: success being defined by the lack of unedifying skirmishes between any of the parties (particularly Robert's parents who are prone that way). Robert's 'Indian' cousin Farzad is about to study international relations at NYU and was an absolute delight to have about. He was good with the children and took our Romanian au-pair, Ioana, out dancing which pleased her. He had the confident, self-possessed, air of many young North Americans, but without the insular world view or right wing politics (his family moved from Bombay to the States when he was twelve). So we were a really international melting-pot family this Christmas with Eilish's Scottish/ French ancestry in addition to my own Irish/English roots; Jacquie grew up in German speaking Zurich and Rumy in Bombay speaking Gujarati (but the Parsis celebrate Christmas too, just for good measure). Then we had the young dashing North American just to top things off.

***

I didn't look at the television on Boxing Day or subsequently, so I was unaware of the Tsunami and the rising death toll. Later, I heard some moving reportage on the radio stating that in some of the worst affected areas many thousands more women then men were drowned; speculation about this fact given was that men are stronger swimmers than women, but also that many women drowned trying to save their babies and children. I can imagine not letting go of my children.

Thursday 30th Dec 04.

I've realised why I am experiencing such a strong emotional resistance to finishing this book, and it's a book-length book now so there is no reason to keep writing: I won't have a baby if I stop. While I am writing this diary I might still conceive. After all, this is a *conception* dairy. This kind of thinking is utterly irrational, of course. I can stop writing this diary right now and in a month or a year I might be pregnant, but it doesn't *feel* like that. I am having difficulty letting go. My desire to have another baby fluctuates in intensity but it remains: like a heartbeat, like a breath; when I am quiet I become aware of it. Finishing this book means turning my back on that wish, and starting a new phase of my life. I fear, after almost two years of 'trying to have a baby', that I am too old – there, I've said it.

Friday 31st December 05.
It's New Year's Eve and I can say with sincerity that Robert and I are happier now than at any other point in the year. We have reached a point of calm. I'm feeling very slightly peaky – something I ate I suspect but, of course, part of me is watching carefully for the early conception nausea which I now long to experience.

Saturday 1st January 05.
I feel this conception diary is coming to an end. I am no longer convinced that I shall ever have a third child. I have tried and failed. I may be able to add a post-script, but I am beginning to suspect that I may not. I am one of the many professional women who had children too late in life; by the time we realised what a joy children are, we find that we are unable to conceive.

I feel good about being a mother and it is undoubtedly the most meaningful part of my life. But the reality of today is that women cannot compete with men in the workplace, or in the public sphere in general, unless they are childless. In the present climate you have got to be able to work unsocial hours, or be prepared to move to take up opportunities in another town, or country, for advancement: to 'relocate', and how many women can drag around two or three or four children and a spouse? The answer is, not many.

Notes

March 5th. Lucy Cavendish *`Loneliness, tears and the shock of the new NHS'* London Standard. 1st March 03.

March 21st. Carol Shields. 2002. Unless. London: Fourth Estate.

April 3rd. Owen Bowcott *`Iraqis Firing From Shrine'* (piece on checkpoint shooting). The Guardian. Thursday 3rd April 03. p. 2.

April 4th. Jen Marshall. 2002. *Crossing to Saftey* p.63 in Hanauser, C. (ed.) The Bitch in the House. London: Penguin, Viking.

April 5th. Rory McCarthy. *`Car bomb kills three soldiers and two Iraqis at checkpoint'.* The Guardian. Saturday April 5th, 2003. p.3.

May 19th. Lucy Cavendish. *'Curse of the Mummy. Mothers and childcare gurus are on the warpath... and there're all after Lucy Cavendish'.* The Observer Review. (Living).18 May 2003. p.4.

June 1st. Emma Loach. *'The Hardest Thing I have Ever Done'* The Guardian Weekend. 31.05.03. p.32-37.

June 14th. The buggy is a Land rover.

June 14st 03. *`Court Win for Fathers in MMR Jabs Fight'.* Saturday Guardian. p. 2.

June 25th 03. Hewlett, S. A. 2002. Baby Hunger: The New Battle for Motherhood. London: Atlantic Books. p.91. High achievement is defined as $55,000 or $65,000 depending on age. Ultras achievers ate on $100,000.

July 4th 03. Advertisement for a research programme. Times Higher Educational Supplement. p.49.

July 10th 03. Thomas, P. *'Money Running Out for Convenience Caesareans'.* Aims Journal. Vol. 14. No. 3. pp.1-2.

June 20th 03. Hinsliff, G. *'War Zone' NHS Drives Women to Home Births.* The Observer. News. p.8.

August 30. 03. Bennett, C. and Fishel, S. *'When All You Want is a Baby'* The Guardian. Comment and Analysis. p.24.

September 13. 03. Briscoe, J. '*The Generation That Took a Gamble*'. The Guardian Weekend. pp.21-28.

September 14. 03. Barbara Ellen. *Tiny Feat.* Observer Magazine. pp.23-28.

September 16th – James Meikle. '*New hi-tech scans show babies smiling and crying before birth'.* The Guardian. National News. Saturday

September 13th 2003. p.5.

September 4th 03. Cusk, R. *'Darkness at the Heart of the Family'* [Cusk talks to Shriviner about her novel *We Need to Talk About Kevin*] in The Guardian Weekend. 04.10.03. pp.45-50.

October 10th 03. Zoe Williams. *The Parent Trap*. Guardian Weekend Magazine. 18.10.03. pp.60-64.

October 19th 03. Rose Shepherd. *Happily Unblessed*. OM. The Observer Magazine. Real Lives. 19.10.03. pp.48-54.

December 28th 03. Comment. *Let's Put Women and Children First*. The Observer. 28.12.03. p.24.

January 11th 04. O'Keeffe, A. *It's a Tough Call – But Should She Have to Make it?* The Observer Focus : Equality at Work. 11. 01. 04. p.20.

January 18th 04. Anne Moore. *Mother's Ruin*. OM. The Observer Magazine. Real Lives. 18.01.04. pp. 34-39.

January 25th 04. Simms, S. *What Happened Next?* OM. The Observer Magazine. Life. 25.01.04. p.86.

Febrauary 7th 04. Bindel, J. *It's a Family Affair*. Guardian Weekend. 07.02.04. p. 7.

February 15th 04. Laura Ashton and Anushka Asthana. Nappies *at Fifty.* The Observer Focus. Older Mothers. p. 19.

March 13th 04. Suzanne Goldenberg. *'Caesarean refusal' mother in jail.* The Observer. News. p.2.

March 20th 04.: Helen Carter. *'Mother on drinking binge left baby in car'.* The Guardian, News. p.13.

March 20th 04.: Suzanne Goldenberg. *'Baby given eight new organs in record transplant*. The Guardian, News. p.2.

March 20th 04.: Kate Figes & Ellie Lee. *Mother's ruin* (e-mail debate). The Guardian. Comment and Analysis. p.24.

May 2nd 2004. Anna Moore. *Why Choice is our Birthright: A Mother's Tale*. The Observer. Focus. p. 18.

&

May 2nd 2004. Nicholas Fisk and Sara Patterson Brown. *The Safest Method of Birth is by Caesarean Section: A Doctor's Tale*. The Observer. Focus. p. 18.

May 23rd. 2004. Jo Revil & Judy Hobson. *Increase in attacks on pregnant women*. The Observer. News. p. 4.

May 23rd. 2004. David Aaronovich. *Why dads throw flour*. The Observer. Comment. p..29.
June 6th. 2004. Lisa O'Kelly. *It Beats Working*. The Observer. Review. p. 1-2.
June 13th 2004. Kathryn Flett. *The mother of all rows*. The Observer. Living. p. 4.
June 26th 2004. Rachel Shabi. *Baby Chase*. The Guardian Weekend. pp. 14-23.
17th July 2004. Rebecca Abrams. *Minding the Baby. Why Love Matters: How Affection Shapes a Baby's Brain*. The Guardian Review. Book of the Week. p.9.
1st August 2004. Vanessa Thorpe. *No Going Back.* A review of *Making Babies: Stumbling into Motherhood* by Anne Enright. The Observer Review. p.16.
14th August 2004. Rebecca de Saintonge. *No Kidding*. The Guardian Weekend. pp.20-23.
10th September 2004. Peter Conrad. *Should We Have Looked Away?* Review. The Observer. p. 1-2.
14th September 2004. Cole, Babette. 1993. Mummy Laid an Egg! London: Radom House. ISBN: 0 09 9299119.
18th September 2004. Literary Review. *Birth Pains*. Review of Anne Enright's Making Babies in Private Eye. p.24.
18th October 04.
Edmund, M. 1994. *A Bitter Political Pill* in Dying to Have a Baby. A supplement produced by The Observer; Marie Stopes International & Interact Worldwide. p.14.
&
George, S. 1994. *What's Going On?* A supplement produced by The Observer; Marie Stopes International & Interact Worldwide. p.4.
24th October 04. Groskop, V. 1994. *Why I wish I'd been a young mum*. The Observer. Focus: The Baby Controversy. p.20.

Acknowledgements (copyright):
'Iraqis Firing From Shrine', 'Iraqis Firing From Shrine' Owen Bowcott, The Guardian. 3/4/2003. Copyright Guardian Newspapers Limited 2003; Jen Marshall. 2002. *Crossing to Safety* p.63 in Hanauser, C. (ed.) The

Bitch in the House. London: Penguin, Viking. Thanks to Harper Colins, U.K.; *'Car bomb kills three soldiers and two Iraqis at checkpoint.'* Rory McCarthy, The Guardian. 5/4/ 2003. Copyright Guardian Newspapers Limited 2003; *'Curse of the Mummy. Mothers and childcare gurus are on the warpath... and there're all after Lucy Cavendish'* Lucy Cavendish, The Observer Review. 18/5/03. Copyright Guardian Newspapers Limited 2003; 'The *Hardest Thing I have Ever Done'*, Emma Loach, The Guardian Weekend. 31/05/2003. Copyright Guardian Newspapers Limited 2003; '*Court Win for Fathers in MMR Jabs Fight',* No author listed, Saturday Guardian. 2/06/2003. Copyright Guardian Newspapers Limited 2003; *'War Zone' NHS Drives Women to Home Births'.* G. Hinsliff, G. The Observer. 20/06/2003. Copyright Guardian Newspapers Limited 2003; *'When All You Want is a Baby',* C. Bennett., S. Fishel, The Guardian. 30/08/2003. Copyright Guardian Newspapers Limited 2003; '*The Generation That Took a Gamble*', J. Briscoe, The Guardian Weekend. 13/09/2003. Copyright Guardian Newspapers Limited 2003; *'Tiny Feat'*, Barbara Ellen, Observer Magazine. 14/09/2003. Copyright Guardian Newspapers Limited 2003; '*New hi-tech scans show babies smiling and crying before birth',* James Meikle, The Guardian. 13/09/2003. Copyright Guardian Newspapers Limited 2003; *'Darkness at the Heart of the Family', Rachael Cusk,* The Guardian Weekend. 4/10/2003. Copyright Guardian Newspapers Limited 2003; 'The *Parent Trap',* Zoe Williams, The Guardian Weekend. 18/10/2003. Copyright Guardian Newspapers Limited 2003;*'Happily Unblessed',* Rose Shepherd, The Observer Magazine. 19/10/2003. Copyright Guardian Newspapers Limited 2003;*'Let's Put Women and Children First'*, No author listed, The Observer. 28/12/2003. Copyright Guardian Newspapers Limited 2003;*'It's a Tough Call – But Should She Have to Make it?', A.* O'Keeffe, The Observer. 11/01/2004. Copyright Guardian Newspapers Limited 2004; *'Mother's Ruin',* Anne Moore, The Observer Magazine. 18/01/2004. Copyright Guardian Newspapers Limited 2004; *'What Happened Next?*', S. Simms. The Observer Magazine. 25/01/04. Copyright Guardian Newspapers Limited 2004; *'It's a Family Affair',* J. Bindel, Guardian Weekend. 07/02/2004. Copyright Guardian Newspapers Limited 2004; *'Nappies at Fifty',* Laura Ashton and Anushka Asthana, The Observer. 15/02/2004. Copyright Guardian Newspapers Limited

2004; *'Caesarean Refusal' Mother in Jail'*, Suzanne Goldenberg, The Observer. 13/03/2004. Copyright Guardian Newspapers Limited 2004; *'Mother on Drinking Binge Left Baby in Car'*, Helen Carter, The Guardian. 20/03/2004. Copyright Guardian Newspapers Limited 2004; *'Baby Given Eight New Organs in Record Transplant'*, Suzanne Goldenberg, The Guardian. 20/03/2004. Copyright Guardian Newspapers Limited 2004; *'Mother's Ruin'*, Kate Figes & Ellie Lee, The Guardian. 20/03/2004. Copyright Guardian Newspapers Limited 2004; *'Why Choice is our Birthright: A Mother's Tale'*, Anna Moore, The Observer. 02/05/2004. Copyright Guardian Newspapers Limited 2004; *'The Safest Method of Birth is by Caesarean Section: A Doctor's Tale'*, The Observer. 02/05/2004. Copyright Guardian Newspapers Limited 2004; *'Increase in Attacks on Pregnant Women'*, Jo Revil & Judy Hobson, The Observer. 23/05/2004. Copyright Guardian Newspapers Limited 2004; *'Why Dads Throw Flour'*, David Aaronovich, The Observer. 23/05/2004. Copyright Guardian Newspapers Limited 2004; *'It Beats Working'*, Lisa O'Kelly. The Observer. 6/06/2004. Copyright Guardian Newspapers Limited 2004; *'The Mother of All Rows'*, Kathryn Flett, The Observer. 13/06/2004. Copyright Guardian Newspapers Limited 2004; *'Baby Chase'*, Rachel Shabi, The Guardian Weekend. 26/06.2004. Copyright Guardian Newspapers Limited 2004; *'Minding the Baby. Why Love Matters: How Affection Shapes a Baby's Brain'*, Rebecca Abrams, The Guardian Review. 17/06/2004. Copyright Guardian Newspapers Limited 2004; *'No Going Back.* A review of *Making Babies: Stumbling into Motherhood* by Anne Enright', The Observer Review. 1/08/2004. Copyright Guardian Newspapers Limited 2004; *'No Kidding'*, Rebecca de Saintonge, The Guardian Weekend. 14/09/2004. Copyright Guardian Newspapers Limited 2004; *Should We Have Looked Away?,* Peter Conrad, The Observer. 10/09/2004. Copyright Guardian Newspapers Limited 2004; *'Birth Pains'*, No author. Private Eye. 18/09/2004; Copyright Private Eye; *'A Bitter Political Pill'*, M Edmund, Dying to Have a Baby. 18/10/2004. Copyright Guardian Newspapers Limited 2004; *'What's Going On?'*, S. George , Dying to Have a Baby. 18/10/2004. Copyright Guardian Newspapers Limited 2004; *'Why I Wish I'd Been a Young Mum'*, V. Groskop, The Observer. 14/10/2004. Copyright Guardian Newspapers Limited 2004;